THE
UNCERTAIN NERVOUS SYSTEM

THE UNCERTAIN NERVOUS SYSTEM

by

B. DELISLE BURNS

Head of the Division of Physiology and Pharmacology
National Institute for Medical Research, London, England,
formerly Professor of Physiology
McGill University, Montreal, Canada

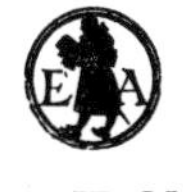

LONDON

EDWARD ARNOLD (PUBLISHERS) LTD

First published 1968

SBN: 7131 4125 5

Printed in Great Britain by
The Camelot Press Ltd., London and Southampton

PREFACE

AUTHORS frequently preface academic publications with a selection of altruistic phrases; reference is often made to the long-felt need for such a work, to the timely filling of an intellectual gap. It would be hypocrisy for me to make any statement of this sort, for I wrote the pages that follow primarily for my own amusement. Like many people, I think more clearly in the presence of an audience; I reach a conclusion more rapidly when I talk or write. Consequently, I wrote this book largely in order to define my own beliefs and to specify a little more clearly a few working hypotheses that might guide my own research. Nevertheless, one cannot write without having some particular audience in mind.

The result is a monograph which stresses the inter-disciplinary nature of central neurophysiology, a subject in which progress has come to depend upon some knowledge of classical physiology, experimental psychology, applied mathematics and electronic engineering. Since I am not an expert in all these fields, I have been forced to think and write in relatively simple terms. Thus, although this is a technical book, mainly concerned with the problems of contemporary research, what I have said should prove intelligible and relevant to the interests of final-year undergraduates and postgraduate research students in several disciplines.

Even when a book is published in the name of one author, it usually expresses indirectly the views of many people. My own opinions have been shaped by conversation and correspondence with many friends; I have doubtless conveniently forgotten some of these dialogues and now claim their consequences as the product of my own thoughts. Nevertheless, I am still aware of the general debt that I owe to my graduate students and to the professional scientists who have worked with me.

I began writing this book while spending a year's sabbatical leave at the National Physical Laboratory, Teddington, England. During this time I received a Carnegie Fellowship. Thus, my first specific thanks must go to McGill University, which gave me leave, to the Carnegie Institution, which supported this enterprise and to my host, the Autonomics Division of the National Physical Laboratory.

Parts of the preliminary manuscript have been read and constructively criticized by a number of my friends—who nevertheless cannot be held responsible for the end result! My particular thanks are due to Professor Lloyd Stevenson of Yale, to Professor A. M. Uttley of Sussex, to Drs. Grant Smith and Roy Pritchard of McMaster and to Drs. T. V. P. Bliss and George Mandl of McGill.

I have not been able to resist frequent reference to my own research work. Consequently, while writing, I have been often reminded of my indebtedness to McGill University, which provided the necessary space and time for my work, and to both the Canadian Medical Research Council and Canadian Defence Research Board which provided the tools. These three organizations gave me all the encouragement that I needed during sixteen enjoyable and stimulating years spent in Canada.

Writing the first draft of a book or paper is an enjoyable and carefree occupation. One can misquote rival authors, sketch barely intelligible diagrams in pencil and make one's hypotheses more credible by underlining them. It is when the first draft is complete that the really hard work begins—the correction of references, the drawing and photography of persuasive diagrams, the conversion of an illegible manuscript into elegant type. In this again I was given willing help by many people. Mr. Klaus Fabich made and photographed many of the figures in these pages. For the tedious work of typing and retyping, I am indebted to Miss M. Standish, Miss K. O'Rourke and Mrs. J. Hunt. Lastly I must thank the publishers for their painstaking preparation of the final product.

October, 1967 B. DELISLE BURNS

CONTENTS

CHAPTER 1

ANALOGUES FOR THE NERVOUS SYSTEM

History of analogues for the nervous system

The functions of the brain and spinal cord have usually been described in terms that were borrowed from the study of some well-known communications system. Thus, the brain was once believed to be the central reservoir of a complex hydraulic machine, which permitted the periodic flow of vital spirits into the muscles (Foster, 1901). It was known that skeletal muscles were paralysed when their nerve supply was cut and it was consequently assumed that the central nervous system governed their activity through the muscular nerves. But the nature of the invisible message that travelled down these nerve trunks was uncertain. The facts could apparently be explained by assuming that nerve trunks were made from many fine tubes, down which the central nervous system pumped a fluid that distended the muscles. Thus, it seemed that joints were moved by inflation of the appropriate muscles with vital spirits from the central nervous system; an inflation which anyone can see who watches a strong man flex his elbow against a load. "In proportion as the animal spirits enter the cavities of the brain, they pass thence into the pores of its substance, and from these pores into the nerves; where according as they enter, more or less, into this or that nerve, they have the power of changing the shape of the muscles into which the nerves are inserted, and by this means making all the limbs move. Thus, as you may have seen in the grottoes and fountains in our gardens, the force with which water issues from its reservoir is sufficient to put into motion various machines. . . . These animal spirits are like a wind or a very subtle flame. . . . And though they are very subtle and lively, yet when they flow into a muscle they cause it to become stiff and swollen, just as the air in a balloon makes it hard and stretches the substance in which it is contained" (Descartes, 1664).

This hypothesis remained tenable until Glisson demonstrated in the seventeenth century that the volume of active muscle was less than that of resting muscle. "But indeed this explosion and inflation of spirits has now for some time past been silenced, convicted by the following experiment. Take an oblong glass tube of suitable capacity and shape. Fit into the top of its side near its mouth another small tube like a funnel. Let a strong muscular man insert into the mouth of the larger tube the whole of his bared arm, and secure the mouth of the tube all round to the humerus with bandages so that no water can escape from the tube. . . . It will be seen that when the muscles are contracted the water in the tube of the funnel sinks, rising again when relaxation takes place. . . . From this therefore we may infer that the fibres are shortened by an intrinsic vital movement and have no need of any afflux of spirits, either animal or vital, by which they are inflated, and being so shortened carry out the movements ordered by the brain." (Translation from Glisson's *De Ventriculo* (1677) by Foster, 1901.)

Glisson had discovered facts that were inconsistent with current beliefs; his arguments would have been more persuasive, however, had he been able to offer a satisfactory alternative hypothesis. The result is that we find Alexander Monro (1763) writing of Glisson's observation in a textbook for medical students some ninety years later, "To this it has been answered. . . . That the spaces between the muscular fibres are sufficient to lodge these fibres when they swell, during the contraction of a muscle, without any addition to its bulk; and that it plainly appears that these spaces between the fibrils are thus occupied, by the compression which the larger vessels of muscles, which run in those spaces, suffer during the action of the muscle; it is so great as to drive the blood in the veins with a remarkable accelerated velocity."

The nature of the nervous message was to remain a mystery until the discovery of electricity.

It is no longer fashionable to liken the nervous system to an hydraulic arrangement of reservoirs and fine tubes. Since the time of Descartes, physiologists have found other more useful terms in which to describe nervous function; nevertheless, these were still concepts borrowed from some contemporary, man-made system of communication. For a time, each analogy has served its function of simplifying description and furthering knowledge by suggesting new experiments, and has then been deserted for a better set of hypotheses. No doubt, the descriptions of nervous function that we find adequate today will seem laughable to the patronizing historian of 2067. "For indeed, it is one of the lessons of the history of science that each age steps on the shoulders of the ages that have gone before. The value of each age is not its own, but is in part, in large part, a debt to its forerunners. And this age of ours if, like its predecessors, it can boast of something of which it is proud, would, could it read the future, doubtless find also much of which it would be ashamed" (Foster, 1901).

Despite such warnings, one finds that over the years the nervous system has been courageously likened in turn to a collection of water-filled tubes, a telephone exchange consisting of fixed wires and mobile switches, to a collection of self-controlling systems and finally to a man-made general purpose computer. The great value of comparisons of this sort is, of course, that they canalize curiosity and suggest experiments designed to test the extent to which each analogy is tenable. Moreover, in that they point to the similarity between a system with novel and surprising characteristics and one which is 'understood' because it has been frequently encountered, analogies enable one to remember many diverse properties by recalling the one fact of similarity. But there is also danger in this convenient method of classifying information. History shows that the more successful analogies are likely to become interpreted too literally by converts whose faith leads them to confuse likeness with identity. The similarity between the nervous system and a telephone exchange has led some to look for an operator—to seek the "mode of operation of 'will' upon the cerebral cortex" (Eccles, 1953), or the 'site of consciousness' (Penfield & Erickson, 1941). Walshe (1948) has aptly described the latter pursuit as "anatomising an abstraction".

Despite the obvious danger of analogy, it seems that man can only understand by creating models or seeking likenesses in his environment. Even a mathematical formula is a type of model. If I state that the relationship between conduction velocity (V) and axon diameter (D) of myelinated nerve fibres is given by:

$$V = a + b \cdot D$$

(where a and b are constants), I am stressing the parallel between two aspects of the behaviour of nerve and, say, two properties of a tea-pot, for which there is also a rectilinear relationship between the depth of water contained and the rate of overflow from the spout. But there are few other ways in which a nerve is like a tea-pot.

On the other hand, I might assert that nerve fibres behave like a fuse or trail of gunpowder. This statement admittedly lacks the precision of a mathematical equation, but is in some ways more scientifically productive. A single equation cannot point the way to further research, other than that required to check the range of its veracity. In contrast, the statement that a nerve is like a fuse may lead to many different types of experiment, designed to explore the breadth of the original assertion. Walshe (1948) has said the same thing in another way: "For too many amongst us, also, the inadequate conception that 'science is measurement' and concerns itself with nothing but the metrical has become a thought-cramping obsession, and the more nearly a scientific paper approximates to a long and bloodless caravan of equations plodding across the desert pages of some journal between small infrequent oases of words, the more quintessentially scientific it is supposed to be, though not seldom no one can tell—and few are interested to ask—whither in the kingdom of ordered knowledge the caravan is bound."

Despite the seductive elegance of Walshe's prose, it would be most unwise to belittle the value of quantitative statements in neurophysiology. My intention in the preceding paragraphs has been merely to assess the contribution and the limitations of all aspects of model building. The discussion above seems to lead to two propositions which might be made concerning the usefulness of scientific models:

1. the relevance or truth of a model can be assessed from the correspondence in behaviour of pairs of parameters, chosen to be equivalent;
2. the fertility of a model can be measured as the number of equivalent parameters, predicted but not originally foreseen.

The remainder of this chapter is devoted to a summary and discussion of those analogues which have been used during this century as convenient generalizations about the nervous system.

The central nervous system as a telephone exchange

At the end of the last century Pearson (1900) wrote the following passage: "The view of brain activity here discussed may perhaps be elucidated by comparing the brain to the central office of a telephone exchange, from which wires radiate to the subscribers A, B, C, D, E, F, etc., who are senders, and to W, X, Y, Z, etc., who are receivers of messages. A, having notified the company that he never intends to correspond with anybody but W, his wire is joined to W's, and the clerk remains unconscious of the arrival of the message from A and its dispatch to W, although it passes through his office. (If these wires were connected *outside* the office, we should have an analogy to certain possibilities of reflex action, which arise from sensory and motor nerves being linked before reaching the brain—e.g. a frog's leg will be moved so as to rub an irritated point on its back even after the removal of the brain.) There is indeed no call bell. This corresponds to an instinctive exertion following unconsciously on a sense-impression. Next the clerk finds by experience that B invariably desires to correspond with X, and consequently whenever he hears B's call-bell he links him mechanically to X, without stopping for a moment his perusal of *Tit-Bits*. This corresponds to an habitual exertion following unconsciously on a sense impression. Lastly, C, D, E and F may set their bells ringing for a variety of purposes; the clerk has in each case to answer their demands but this may require him to listen to the special communications of these subscribers, to examine his lists, his Post Office directory, or any other source of information stored in his office. Finally, he shunts their wires so as to bring them in circuit with those of Y and Z, which seem to best suit the nature of the demands. This corresponds to an exertion following consciously on the receipt of a sense-impression."

A telephone system can be constructed from a number of wires converging upon a central switchboard. By the use of prearranged rules, messages conveyed towards the exchange along a particular wire, may be channelled through the switchboard so as to leave the exchange along some other chosen route. It is this concept of a number of sensory channels making fixed connections with a central 'switchboard', which connects input to motor outputs according to complex but unchanging laws, that has proved so useful to an understanding of spinal reflex responses.

It was Sherrington's success in using such ideas that led Pavlov and many others to attempt the description of conditioned reflexes in similar terms. It was argued, I think correctly, that learning must involve a rerouting of excitation within the central nervous system. Before conditioning, the sensory excitation produced by a ringing bell may cause only a turning of the animal's head; after conditioning, the same afferent input to the nervous system can produce the motor response of salivation. It was supposed, therefore, that synaptic junctions within the brain could operate as switches capable of redirecting sensory input into new channels; the setting of these switches would, of course, be determined by the past experience of the nervous system. Thus, while the spinal cord was to be considered as a telephone exchange with relatively fixed connections (in which, for instance, subscriber A was always connected to subscriber N, and output O only occurred in response to simultaneous inputs through A and B), the cerebral cortex provided a similar exchange with more flexible connections between input and output. Connections of the sensory input with the cortical exchange appeared to be fixed in the sense that a particular cortical district was excited by each sensory modality; likewise, localized points of departure for the cortical motor output were demonstrable in the 'motor cortex'. The switching function of cortical synapses presumably constructed channels through which excitation might pass rapidly and easily from the sensory cortex excited by a conditioned stimulus to the appropriate parts of the motor cortex.

This simple concept of learning was severely shaken by Lashley's attempts to find the cortical pathways that had been facilitated when rats were trained (Lashley, 1929). His experiments showed that a specific acquired habit was not diminished as a result of localized cortical injury, as would have been predicted from the unmodified telephone-exchange theory of learning. Admittedly, cortical destruction did interfere with learning ability and retention, but the degree of interference appeared to correlate with the quantity of cortex destroyed rather than the locality of ablation. Lashley has said of the reflex theory of behaviour: "The chief difficulty is its implication of a point-for-point correspondence in the relations of receptors, nerve cells and effectors. Not that this is always expressed; but the comprehensibility and explanatory value of the reflex-arc hypothesis lies in just this definiteness of connections, which permits the tracing of nerve impulses over predetermined paths. Omit this element of restricted paths and the theory becomes nothing more than an assertion of uniformity in the sequence of stimulus and response. . . . The doctrine of isolated reflex conduction has been widely influential in shaping current psychological theories. Its assumptions that reactions are determined by local conditions in limited groups of neurones, that learning consists of the modification of resistance in isolated synapses, that retention is the persistence of such modified conditions, all make for a conception of behaviour as rigidly department-alized."

Moreover, Lashley and others (Hebb, 1949) have often pointed out that the conditioned stimuli used during the formation of a conditioned reflex response, are unlikely to excite exactly the same sensory receptors in any two presentations. It is the pattern of sensory excitation which becomes conditioned, not a series of specific sensory endings, or afferent neurones. With respect to excitation by retinal patterns, Lashley said (1929): "This means that, not only on the retina, but also in the central projection on the cortex, there is a constant flux of stimulation, such that the same cells are rarely, if ever, twice excited by the same stimulus, yet a constant reaction is produced. The activity of the visual cortex must resemble that of one of the electric signs in which a pattern of letters passes rapidly across a stationary group of lamps. The structural pattern is fixed, but the functional pattern plays over it without limitation to specific elements." One is reminded here of the frequently quoted pass-age from Sherrington (1940), which I find more poetic but much less informative. Asking us to imagine activity of neurones as shown by little points of light, he describes the brain as " . . . an enchanted loom where millions of flashing shuttles weave a dissolving pattern, always a mean-ingful pattern though not ever an abiding one; a shifting harmony of sub-patterns".

There seems little reason to believe that the motor response of a con-ditioned reflex involves the same motoneurones in the same sequence on every occasion. Hebb (1949) when discussing 'Motor Equivalence' says "A rat trained to depress a lever to get food may do so from any of several positions, in each of which the muscular pattern is different. He may climb on the lever; press it down with the left forefoot, or the right; or use his teeth instead. Very often, all that can be predicted after the response is learned is that the lever will be moved downward. It is not necessary here to multiply examples of such behaviour; it will be evident to anyone who cares to watch animal or man carry out a learned res-ponse." Many experimental observations are consistent with Hebb's generalization. Monkeys trained to respond in a certain manner by the use of one limb—to open a problem box, for example—will complete the task with the mouth or another limb if the 'trained' limb is temporarily paralysed by localized surgical destruction of its sensory-motor cortex (Lashley, 1924; Jacobsen, 1932; Glees & Cole, 1950).

Moreover, Sperry (1947) has shown that multiple intersecting knife-cuts, perpendicular to the brain's surface and severing the grey matter of the sensory-motor cortex, do not interfere with learned responses of the represented limb, provided that the cuts do not extend into the underlying white matter. Interference with white matter, presumably because of consequent damage to cortico-cortical association fibres, produced a local abolition of learned responses which matched complete cortical excision in its severity.

The weakness of Lashley's argument was similar to that of Glisson in the seventeenth century. Lashley subjected the telephone-exchange or reflex theory of behaviour to quantitative tests and managed to expose its failings without offering any promising set of alternative concepts. When reviewing his own work in 1950 he said: "It is difficult to interpret such findings, but I think that they point to the conclusion that the associative connections or memory traces of the conditioned reflex do not extend across the cortex as well defined arcs or paths. Such arcs are either diffused through all parts of the cortex, presumably by relay through lower centres, or do not exist. . . . I sometimes feel, in reviewing the evidence on the localization of the memory trace, that the necessary conclusion is that learning just is not possible." (Lashley, 1950)

Self-controlling systems

Surrounded as one is today with man-made self-controlling systems, it is easy to see that many of the results of behavioural studies described above would have seemed far easier to understand if some use could have been made of cybernetic concepts. When a conditioned reflex is created, some pattern of sensory excitation acquires the property of setting up an unstable state in the nervous system; a state of unrest, which persists until some goal is achieved. It is the relation between sensory pattern and goal which is constant, not the relation between excitation of specific sensory endings and specific motoneurones. Clearly, there is a similarity between the behaviour of a household refrigerator and that of an animal executing a learned task. Figure 1 is intended to illustrate this analogy. The 'flow-diagram' is shown in Fig. 1a. (The closed loop of arrows is often referred to as a 'feed-back' loop around which 'information' may flow.) In Fig. 1b a similar diagram is sketched for a less conventional refrigerator that would learn to behave like the cheaper model above, by a process of trial and error. The 'trial-and-error' switch is supposed to programme the instrument for a number of possible 'motor acts', such as turning off the refrigerator light, switching off the power to the motor, etc., the majority of which would have little effect upon internal temperature. The machine would rapidly learn to behave like the more conventional, pre-programmed model illustrated in Fig. 1a. (Incidentally, by the addition of a 'proprioceptive' element in the door, or an 'eye', which might be supplied as accessories, the instrument could rapidly learn to activate its motor whenever someone opened the door, or approached the refrigerator.)

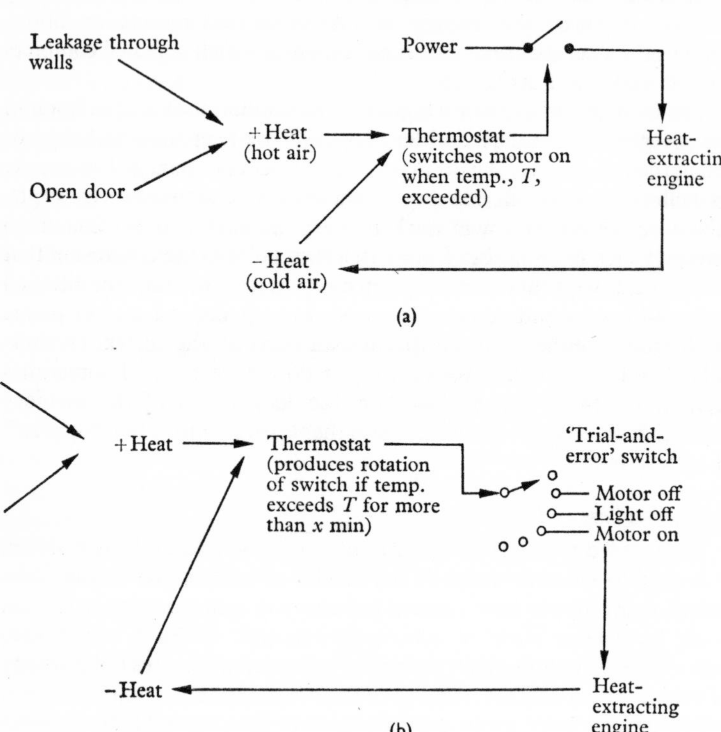

FIG. 1. Self-controlling systems: (*a*) conventional household refrigerator; (*b*) a refrigerator that would learn.

There seems little doubt that a consideration of the properties of self-controlling machines would have helped Lashley out of some of his conceptual difficulties. For instance, the performance of self-controlling machines is relatively insensitive to damage of their parts. A household refrigerator will maintain a constant temperature, even if the heat-extracting engine becomes mechanically less efficient. Had we provided the machine of Fig. 1b with several different mechanisms for extracting heat from the internal air, it would still have learned to control its own temperature. Subsequent damage to a fraction of these heat-extracting mechanisms would not impair its acquired behaviour. Such an instrument, damaged in this way, would be slower to learn, and having learned would react more slowly than the undamaged machine. In fact, it would in many ways show functional deficits similar to those seen in experimental rats with damaged brains.

A hungry animal can be described as a goal-seeking machine which remains in a state of instability until its hunger is satisfied. This instability of the nervous system will be increased by the sight of food or by the provision of a conditioned stimulus. Thus, one can regard the conditioned stimulus as having acquired the ability to set up, or increase, an unstable state of the nervous system, of which salivation forms a part. In terms of Fig. 1, providing a trained animal with a conditioned stimulus is similar to increasing the sensitivity of the thermostat, or reducing its hysteresis. Where the refrigeration system had previously remained stable in the presence of a relatively large difference between actual internal air temperature and maximum permitted temperatures, it would suddenly become active until the required minimum temperature was attained. This analogy is illustrated in Fig. 2.

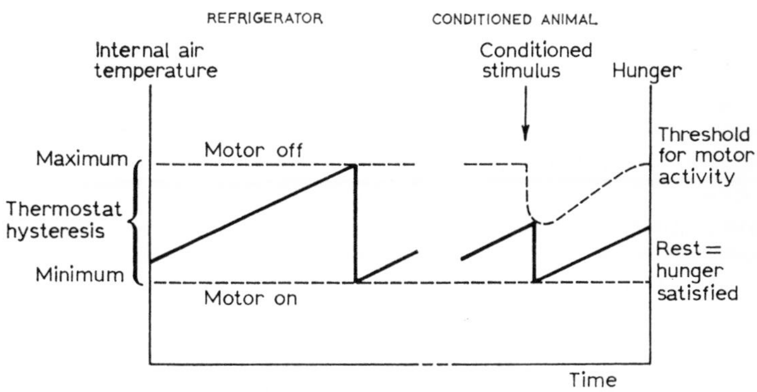

FIG. 2. Illustration of the similarity between a household refrigerator and an animal performing a learned task.

In a similar way one can describe the conditioned stimulus for an avoidance response as creating an unstable state in a nervous system, continually seeking stability and relative inactivity of skeletal muscles. Imagine that an animal (or man) has been taught that the ringing of a bell heralds the administration of a painful stimulus; the latter can be avoided by depressing a spring-loaded switch. When training is complete, the conditioned stimulus sets up instability in the nervous system, producing an unpredictable sequence of motor responses, the only common factor of which is that they terminate once the switch is depressed. Thus, a particular auditory input from the ear can be regarded as having set up a state of instability within a goal-seeking nervous system; the goal in this case being a number of sensory messages informing the nervous system that the switch is depressed. Put in another way, the conditioned stimulus programmes the nervous system for "Motor output until a specific input occurs".

Such statements could be criticized as simply playing with words, for translation of the known facts concerning conditioned reflex formation into a new language cannot increase our knowledge. On the other hand, when described in this way, it becomes clear that a conditioned stimulus creates instability by imposing new conditions for stability—or new stable states. Such similarities with man-made self-controlling instruments justify new questions that might be asked about animal learning. It would seem reasonable, for instance, to search for those mechanisms by which a conditioned stimulus becomes able to set up new conditions for stability within the nervous system. One should perhaps also ask "What is the nature of a stable state in the brain?" Ashby (1952) has given an admirable account of those properties of cybernetic machines most relevant to current neurophysiological problems.

Quite apart from the neurophysiology of learning, there is no doubt concerning the value of cybernetic concepts to the analysis of simpler behavioural problems. For instance, they have successfully been applied (Stark, Campbell & Atwood, 1958; Stark, 1959; Stark, Kupfer & Young, 1965) to an analysis of the reactions of the iris to retinal illumination; Eldred, Granit & Merton (1953) have used them in their interpretation of events in the monosynaptic spinal reflex arc (Granit, 1955; Matthews, 1964). Campbell, Robson & Westheimer (1959) have made use of the same concepts in interpreting accommodation responses of the lens. These and other examples of the biologists' recent use of cybernetic concepts have been reviewed in detail by Milsum (1966).

During the steady viewing of near targets, the refractory power of the human eye undergoes constant fluctuations, implying, of course, a continual contraction and relaxation of the ciliary muscle (Campbell, Robson & Westheimer, 1959). Subjects fixating a target with a large pupil display relatively large oscillations of refractory power at about 2 c/s. This 2 c/s rhythm disappears during distant vision or during observation of an empty field, thus proving that oscillations are dependent upon the presence of changes in sensory feed-back from the retina (Fig. 3). Oscillation about a mean value is a property of all self-controlling systems. For instance, the household refrigerator of Fig. 1 exhibits small fluctuations of internal-air-temperature about a constant mean value that is determined by the setting of the thermostat (Fig. 2). The machine can be described as continually 'hunting' for the correct temperature. The amplitude of these oscillations of temperature is partly dependent upon the sensitivity of the thermostat which controls the instrument. In the case of the human eye viewing a nearby target, the oscillations of refractory power about a mean value, which is 'satisfactory' to the observer, could be regarded as having an origin similar to that producing oscillation of temperature in a household refrigerator.

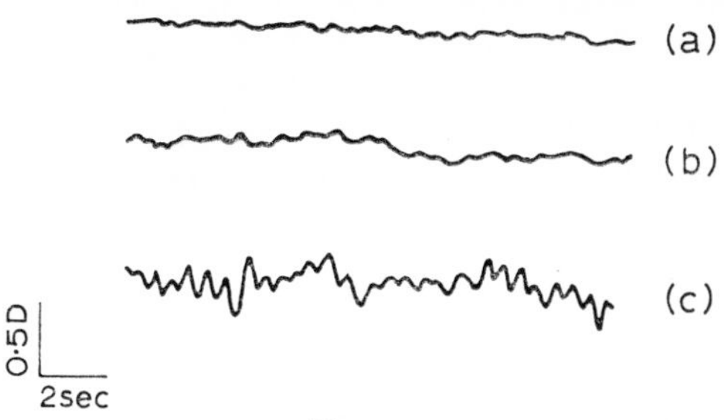

FIG. 3

(*a*) Record of noise generated by optometer with no subject in position.

(*b*) Record while subject J. G. R. viewed a small, high-contrast test object placed at his optical infinity.

(*c*) Record obtained when subject J. G. R. viewed the target placed at 1 D optical distance with a 7 mm pupil.

(From Campbell, Robson & Westheimer, 1959, *J. Physiol*,. **145**, 579, Fig. 2.)

Once a focus of the target's image upon the retina has been achieved which satisfies the nervous system, no further change in motor output to the ciliary muscle is demanded. Sooner or later, however, either a random drift or some other source of instability causes accommodation to become 'unsatisfactory'; presumably the resultant defocusing of the retinal image provides an error signal for the central nervous system which is responsible for readjustment of the ciliary muscle until a satisfactory focus is once again obtained. (Chapter 6 provides some discussion of the central nature of this error signal.) Campbell & Westheimer (1960) have shown that the lens responds to an instantaneous or step-like change of target-range with a time constant of about 0·25 sec. The absence of 2 c/s oscillation when the observer's eye is fixed upon a very distant target will then be due to the absence of significant defocusing with small changes of curvature of the lens; in any case, with distant vision the ciliary muscle is virtually inactive. In some respects, then, the involuntary control of accommodation can be usefully described in terms of a self-controlling reflex in which the information loop or circuit consists of: defocused retinal image; altered behaviour of cortical neurones; modified discharge from motoneurones of the 3rd nerve; contraction or relaxation of ciliary muscle; improved focus of retinal image.

The situation appears, however, to be somewhat more complicated than the above description implies. Campbell, Robson & Westheimer

(1959) found that the oscillation of accommodation disappeared for subjects observing near targets through small pupils. Small pupils give a greater depth of focus than do large pupils; consequently, with contracted pupils one would expect the error signal to be smaller for a given contraction of the ciliary muscle, permitting a greater change in accommodation before correction is initiated. If these were the only factors to be considered, a greater amplitude of oscillation would be expected in subjects viewing through small pupils. In fact, under these conditions, the 2 c/s rhythm disappears (Fig. 4). Campbell *et al.* concluded that "... the simple hypothesis of oscillation through a range of insensitivity cannot be upheld". Nevertheless, their experimental results might be

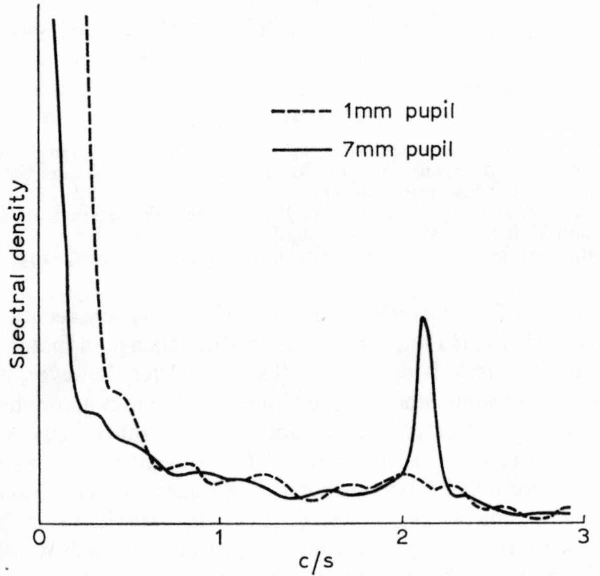

FIG. 4. Frequency spectra for accommodation records of subject J. G. R. under normal viewing conditions with a 7 mm pupil and with a 1 mm effective entrance pupil. The original records showed the same average accommodation level.
(From Campbell, Robson & Westheimer, 1959, *J. Physiol.*, **145**, 579, Fig. 5.)

expected if rate of change of image sharpness formed a significant part of the error signal, as opposed to the absolute degree of defocus.

A similar, but more quantitative analysis, also in terms of a servo-mechanism has proved possible for reactions of the iris to retinal illumination (Stark, Campbell & Atwood, 1958; Stark, 1959; Stark, Kupfer & Young, 1965).

The best-known and perhaps the most successful application of cybernetic concepts in neurophysiological theory originated with Merton's suggestion (1950) that the muscle spindle with its sensory and motor nerves might be an essential element in a reflex servo-mechanism. Muscle spindles are found in every skeletal muscle of the body; each spindle consists of a small fusiform bundle of specialized muscle cells, complete with motor nerve supply. Until recently, however, physiological interest was concentrated upon the sensory nerves which lead from sensory endings within the spindle to the spinal cord. These afferent fibres provide information about muscle length; their discharge frequency is increased by passive stretch of the muscle and is decreased by the active contraction of extrafusal, striated fibres. There appear to be two types of length detector: the 'primary' endings respond to muscle stretch by signalling both the instantaneous length of the muscle and the velocity at which it is being stretched; there also are 'secondary' endings which indicate the instantaneous length without accommodation (Fig. 5). Prior to 1951 it had usually been assumed that the function of the

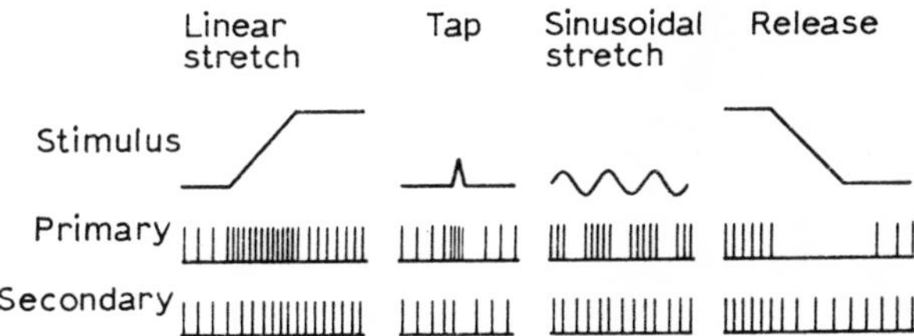

FIG. 5. Diagrammatic comparison of the responses of 'typical' primary and secondary endings to various stimuli. The drawings are based on the reviewer's personal observations as well as those in the literature. The responses are drawn as if the muscle were under moderate initial stretch and as if there were no fusimotor activity.
(From Matthews, 1964, *Physiol. Rev.*, **44**, 245, Fig. 2.)

small motoneurones (γ-motoneurones) innervating intrafusal muscle fibres was to 'take up the slack' and thereby maintain sensitivity of the intrafusal sensory ending during contraction of the surrounding striated fibres. It was known, for instance, that the discharge of γ-motoneurones paralleled that in neighbouring α-motoneurones in all reflex responses except the stretch reflex, during which small nerve discharge was inhibited (Hunt, 1951). For this reason, Kuffler, Hunt & Quilliam (1951) said: "Since the small nerve effect acts synergistically with externally applied tension, its activity would enable the same muscle stretch to cause a similar increment of discharge at different initial tensions, thus providing a peripheral adjustment for maintaining the constancy of the reflex arc in the face of different conditions." Or again, Kuffler and Hunt when reviewing their own work (1952) describe the fusimotor fibres as maintaining "... the afferent flow from spindles in spite of a certain amount of mechanical shortening". While this must undoubtedly be one result of the reflex connections of γ-motoneurones, it is now generally agreed that this description is incomplete in some important respects.

As long ago as 1927, Rossi had suggested as a result of histological observations that the fusimotor fibres might reflexly control the tone of skeletal muscle by causing the intrafusal muscle fibres to contract and thus produce a stretch reflex (Granit, 1955). Merton's proposal (1950) was that the muscle spindles and their small motor fibres formed part of a servo-mechanism by which the length of a skeletal muscle could be reflexly set to any required value. The stretch reflex provided a closed loop control circuit in which passive stretch of the muscle produced an excitation of the primary sensory endings of the spindles; this afferent discharge was relayed direct to motoneurones of the same muscle causing contraction of striated fibres and tension in the muscle tending to restore the original length. On this view, the main function of the monosynaptic arc is to maintain a constant length of skeletal muscle despite variations in the applied load; the precise length which is sought by the servo-system would be dictated by γ-motoneurones which control the sensitivity or 'bias' of length detectors within the spindle. Using once again the analogy of a household refrigerator, a change in the activity of small motoneurones would be the equivalent of setting the thermostat to a new temperature. On this view, the main function of small motor fibres is to determine the range of movement, rather than to compensate for the effects of movement upon the sensory endings. In support of this conception, it has been found that discharge of γ-motoneurones often precedes that of α-motoneurones to the same muscle (Eldred, Granit & Merton, 1953; Granit, 1955; Matthews, 1964).

Apparently, sensory information from muscle spindles is relatively unimportant in conscious proprioception. Position sense in the finger joint is grossly impaired by anaesthetizing the digital nerves, although the spindles in the muscles that move the joint have not been interfered with (Provins, 1958); nor do the spindles of the extrinsic muscles of the human eye seem to contribute to an awareness of the direction of gaze (Brindley & Merton, 1960). Whatever its weakness, the description of the monosynaptic reflex arc, together with the γ-efferents as a length-controlling servo-system, has offered a reasonable explanation for the universal distribution of annulo-spiral endings in skeletal muscles. Not only has it increased our understanding of the simplest and probably basic spinal reflex arc, but it offers a promising framework for future interpretation of many of the tremors encountered in neurological practice. The same concept has been usefully employed to explain the exact adjustment of work performed by the respiratory musculature so as to maintain tidal air constant despite alterations in resistance to air flow (McIlroy, Marshall & Christie, 1954; Campbell & Howell, 1963; Sears, 1964).

General purpose computers

Recent articles stressing the similarities between various functions of the brain and the properties of general purpose computers are so numerous that the point scarcely need be stressed here (Minsky, 1961*a*; Feigenbaum & Feldman, 1963; Ashby, 1966). The main present value of these man-made machines lies in their speed of computation. The human brain can perform the same calculations, but takes some 10^6 times longer. Nevertheless, the human nervous system still remains the better computer in some respects (Camras, 1965). A computer programmed to play chess can apparently be beaten by a moderately skilled human opponent. Minsky (1961*b*) has estimated that "... a search of all the paths through the game of checkers (or draughts) involves some 10^{40} move choices; in chess, some 10^{120}." No man-made computer can yet rival human skill or speed at such tasks as character recognition or language translation. Undoubtedly the most impressive feature of the human brian is its flexibility and the comparatively enormous variety of programmes that can be packed into an instrument occupying less than half a cubic foot, and consuming only some 15 watts. This compact and economical instrument contains some 10^{10} neurones; if one regards the synaptic junction between neurones as the important unit, then the brain might be said to contain about 10^{13} logical elements. If, in some respects, the human brain must be regarded as a relatively slow-operating general purpose computer, in other ways man-made computers appear to be like clumsy and inflexible brains. In either case, the similarity of function has proved so impressive that contemporary neurophysiology is rapidly adopting much of the technical jargon used by computer engineers. Sensory or afferent pathways have become 'inputs'; motoneurones have become 'outputs'; a train of action potentials is often referred to as 'digital information'—all within the last ten years.

The description of the brain as a general purpose computer cannot tell one how the brain works, although it can suggest ways in which the central nervous system *might* operate. For instance, Evans & Newman (1964) have recently suggested a testable hypothesis concerning human dreaming, based upon the observation that man-made computers ultimately become cluttered with useless information and routines, which need periodic erasure for optimal operation. Perhaps the most important influence of this currently fashionable analogy is that neurophysiologists are being forced, by contact with the computer engineer and logician, to define their concepts more precisely.

For the moment, physiology is, as usual, a parasitic science, borrowing the terminology and abstractions developed for another field. It is not impossible, however, that the engineer may ultimately learn something from neurophysiology. It is for this reason that the designers of 'electronic brains' keep a watchful eye upon neurophysiological progress concerning the coding by the central nervous system of sensory input, and the biological mechanism responsible for storage or memory.

In conclusion: noisy communication lines

This introductory chapter was not intended to provide comprehensive reviews of the various analogues that physiologists have used as models for their descriptions of the nervous system. These models have been cited only in order to demonstrate the way in which neurophysiological thought has been dependent upon contemporary engineering. With the passage of time, each set of concepts became inadequate and was replaced by a new terminological structure; often these changes were accompanied by a considerable increase in understanding. Clearly, the identification of major changes in outlook is largely a matter of personal taste. While few people would dispute that the conceptual changes listed above were major, there might reasonably be considerable argument about the intellectual value of these changes.

The remainder of this book is concerned with an attempt to estimate the importance of the most recent addition to the concepts used in neurophysiological thinking—the stochastic or indeterminate behaviour of nerve cells.

Until about twenty years ago, most neurophysiological experiments were performed with the anaesthetized nervous system. Even when anaesthetic was not present, as with investigations of spinal reflexes in the decerebrate animal, artificial synchronous excitation of sensory nerve trunks was used, while responses were picked up with gross electrodes, which recorded the spatial average of action potentials from many motoneurones. The results of such experiments led to an impression that the relation between stimulus and response was predictable with absolute certainty. The same afferent stimulus repeated on a number of separate occasions always appeared to produce a response of the same magnitude. Moreover, the reader of spinal reflex literature from Sherrington through to Eccles is somehow left with the impression that the spinal motoneurone never normally discharges unless the experimenter tells it to. These false impressions are clearly the consequence of extrapolating to the normal animal results that were obtained in necessarily artificial circumstances. Anaesthetic, presumably by interference with synaptic conduction (Butler, 1950; Wright, 1954), so reduces the number of effective afferent pathways to any central neurone, that the responses of this neurone to such excitations as can break through the anaesthetic barrier become both larger and more predictable than they would otherwise be.

That anaesthesia can enlarge and simplify the gross responses evoked from cerebral cortex by sensory excitation has been known for some time; an example of this effect is provided in Fig. 6. In Fig. 7 is shown

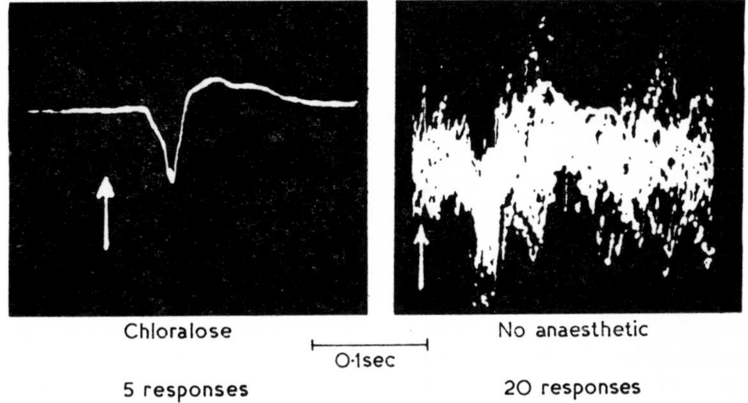

FIG. 6. The standardization of evoked, gross cortical response, produced by chloralose anaesthesia. The stimulus was a brief light flash, given at the arrows. The photographs were obtained by superimposing responses to a number of stimuli.

an effect of light anaesthesia upon the average response of a single neurone in the visual cortex of a cat to excitation of the retina by a flashing source of light. In the case of artificial excitation of the spinal cord, there is no doubt that the stimuli used excite simultaneously many afferent fibres often representing different modalities of sensation, which normally never fire together. This massive synchronous bombardment of central neurones must mask their usual more subtle behaviour; moreover, records made with gross electrodes from ventral roots or from the anterior horn are records of the spatial average of the discharge of many nerve cells, and necessarily hide the whims of individual motoneurones.

In contrast with the types of experiment referred to above, records made with micro-electrodes from single neurones exposed to normal sensory excitation show that the behaviour of neurones in the unanaesthetized central nervous system cannot be predicted with absolute certainty. The first thing that strikes anyone who inserts a micro-electrode into the grey matter of the 'resting' spinal cord in the decerebrate animal, is the large and continual traffic of activity and the essentially unpredictable behaviour of the cells encountered (Fig. 8; Hunt & Kuno, 1959). The same 'spontaneous' activity and a similar stochastic behaviour will be found in both the brain stem and the cerebral cortex. Moreover, responses of single neurones to sensory excitation in the unanaesthetized nervous system are relatively unpredictable in the sense

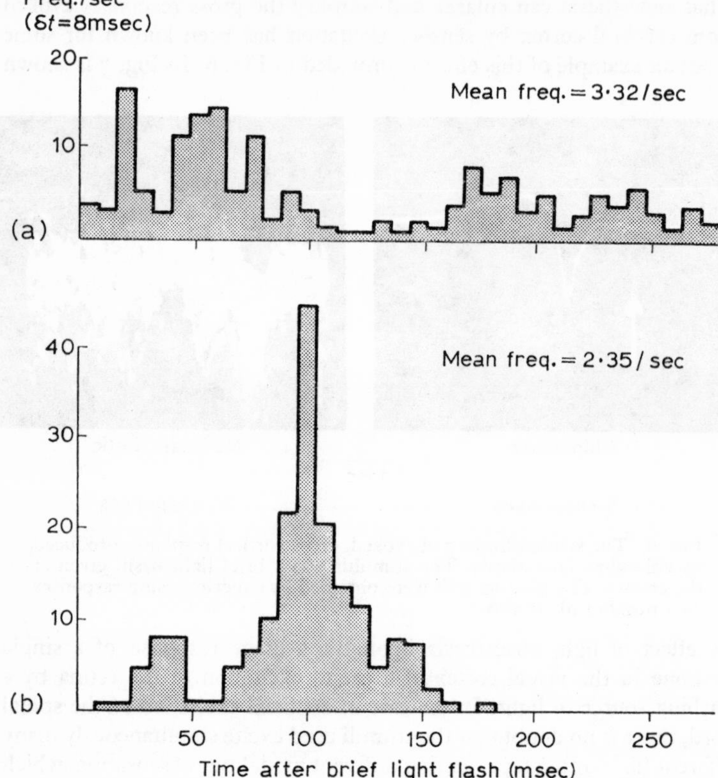

FIG. 7. The effect of light anaesthesia upon the average response of a single neurone in the visual cortex of a cat's isolated fore-brain. The stimulus was a diffuse, brief light flash from a neon bulb, presented to the contralateral retina at 1/sec.

(*a*) The average response to 120 stimuli before anaesthesia.

(*b*) The average response to the same number of stimuli, 20 minutes after giving pentothal (4 mg/kg).

(Personal communication from Mr. A. Robertson.)

that repetition of a series of identical afferent stimuli does not produce a series of identically timed unit responses. A meaningful statement can only be made about the relation between stimulus and response in terms of the *probability* that the unit will respond to the *average* test stimulus. Thus, the response of single neurones to normal sensory excitation is seen superimposed as it were upon the background 'noise' of 'spontaneous activity'—as a signal in a noisy communication system.

This indeterminacy in the response of central neurones is only surprising because one has become so accustomed to the apparent predictability of behaviour derived from older techniques. It is a concept of

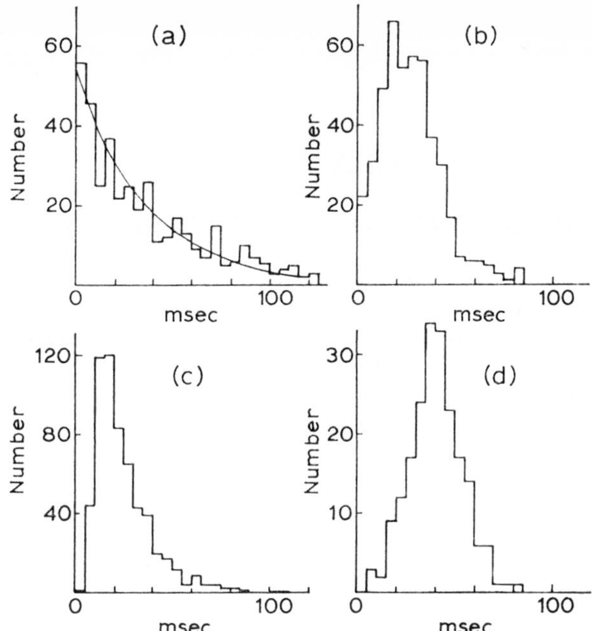

FIG. 8. Frequency distributions of 'spontaneous' impulse intervals in four interneurones (a, b, c, d) characterized by different mean impulse intervals. In (a) the curve represents distribution expected on random basis.
(From Hunt & Kuno, 1959, *J. Physiol.*, **147**, 364, Fig. 2.)

neural activity which is far more likely to be of use to the experimental psychologist, the neurologist and others interested in behaviour of the whole animal. I am, after all, an unpredictable machine; if you call "Burns", there is a high probability that I shall turn my head in your direction—but the probability is always less than unity; my response to this stimulus is not wholly predictable.

It is, then, the stochastic nature of the behaviour of central neurones which forms the main theme of this book. In the chapters which follow, I have tried to show the way in which this new concept has naturally developed as a result of experimental findings, how it has forced the neurophysiologist to use new techniques of analysis and new instruments. The applications of this way of thinking to such problems as 'the spontaneous discharge of central neurones', 'the nature of sensory messages' and 'the physiology of learning' are illustrated. More important perhaps than the application of probability theory to the various restricted fields of neurophysiology referred to below, is the attempt to assess the usefulness and failings of this new concept and the techniques upon which it rests.

CHAPTER 2

PROBABILITY IN PERIPHERAL SYSTEMS

UNTIL 1950, the behaviour of the peripheral nervous system appeared to be completely predictable. Provided that the experimental conditions were carefully controlled, the same stimuli always seemed to produce identical responses. When this was not so, biologists retreated behind such apologetic terms as fatigue, deterioration or tachyphilaxis; in any case, variations in response under apparently constant conditions were not random with respect to time, and statistical analysis was rarely necessary in the analysis of results. Faith in the commendable reliability of peripheral events was finally shaken by the development of the microrecording pipette (Ling & Gerard, 1949), the use of which enabled Fatt & Katz (1951) to examine details of behaviour at the neuromuscular junction.

Miniature end-plate potentials

The discharge of an α-motoneurone in the spinal cord sweeps down the myelinated axon to invade all of its terminal branches; at the end of each of these branches, the end-plates of the nerve terminals, a small quantity of acetylcholine is liberated, which is normally more than sufficient to induce an action potential in the attached muscle fibre. In this way, the whole family of skeletal fibres innervated by one motoneurone contracts whenever the latter discharges. In the rested, normal nerve-muscle preparation, one nerve action potential invariably causes one action potential of each muscle fibre. When such a nerve-muscle preparation is treated with any drug which interferes with neuromuscular transmission by, say, obstructing the access of acetylcholine to the end-plate region of the muscle fibre, the skeletal fibres can only respond to nerve excitation with a local depolarization, restricted to the end-plate region and insufficient to cause a spreading action potential with resulting contraction. This local response to nerve excitation was first observed by Schaefer & Haass (1939) in muscle poisoned with curare and has received considerable attention subsequently (Eccles & O'Connor, 1939; Eccles & Kuffler, 1941; Kuffler, 1943; Fatt, 1950; Fatt & Katz, 1951; Eccles, 1953; Thesleff, 1960). In curarized muscle, the magnitude of the end-plate potential recorded with an intracellular micropipette depends upon the amount of curare present; if it exceeds some 20 mV, or roughly one-fifth of the resting membrane potential of the muscle fibre, conduction will result (Fatt & Katz, 1951).

In 1950, Katz and Fatt first reported evidence of randomly-timed local depolarizations which could be recorded at the end-plate region of frogs' skeletal muscle fibres with an intracellular micropipette when the motor nerves of the preparation were inactive (Katz & Fatt, 1950).

This biological noise in the resting preparation was described as being "... a random succession of miniature end-plate potentials, their amplitude being of the order of 1/100 of the normal end-plate response to a motor nerve impulse" (Fatt & Katz, 1952). They appeared as a series of signals, usually of constant amplitude, occurring at unpredictable times, with a mean frequency between 1–100/sec; this mean frequency was found to increase with increase of temperature and small increases in osmotic pressure. Such variation in amplitude as was observed, appeared to be quantal as though occasionally two or three single units had occurred 'simultaneously' and had added algebraically. Apart from the fact that they could be recorded in the unstimulated nerve-muscle preparation and were very small, these spontaneous local depolarizations had all the appearance of end-plate potentials in curarized muscle. They were made smaller still by the addition of curare; their magnitude and duration were increased by the administration of anticholinesterases (which reduce the normal rate of destruction of acetylcholine by the cholinesterase resident at the muscle end-plate region). Subsequent work by Katz and his collaborators has shown that miniature end-plate potentials are due to a random release by the nerve terminal of quantal packets containing some thousands of acetylcholine molecules (Birks & MacIntosh, 1957; Fatt, 1959; Katz, 1962).

The random release of quanta, referred to above, implies that the escape of a standard packet of acetylcholine is equally likely to occur within any chosen time interval; the chance of escape of each quantum is in no way dependent upon the times of discharge of previous quanta. It can be shown (Feller, 1950) for a series of events with these properties that:

$$n = N \, . \, \delta t/T \, . \, \mathrm{Exp}\,(-t/T)$$

where n = the number of intervals between signals which are more than t and less than $t+\delta t$

N = the total number of signals in a record of duration T.

Fatt and Katz determined the distribution of intervals shown by their records of spontaneous miniature end-plate potentials, and obtained results consistent with the formula given above (Fatt & Katz, 1952).

The normal end-plate potential resulting from nerve stimulation is some 100 times larger than the spontaneous miniature end-plate potentials. Normal transmission from nerve to muscle fibres can be prevented by either increasing the concentration of magnesium ions or decreasing the concentration of calcium ions in the surrounding fluid; unlike curare, these manoeuvres block by reducing the ability of an action potential to release acetylcholine when it arrives at the nerve terminal. Despite the dramatic effect that these ionic changes have upon the release of acetylcholine by a motor nerve, their effect upon the spontaneous release of acetylcholine is small; the frequency of quantal depolarizations is virtually unaltered, while the magnitude of each unit is reduced to some 60% of its normal value (Castillo & Katz, 1954). By reducing in this way the local response of muscle to excitation through its motor nerve to almost vanishing proportions, Castillo and Katz were able to show that the residual response was quantal in nature. Its magnitude was always an integral number of times the size of a spontaneously-occurring miniature end-plate potential (Fig. 9).

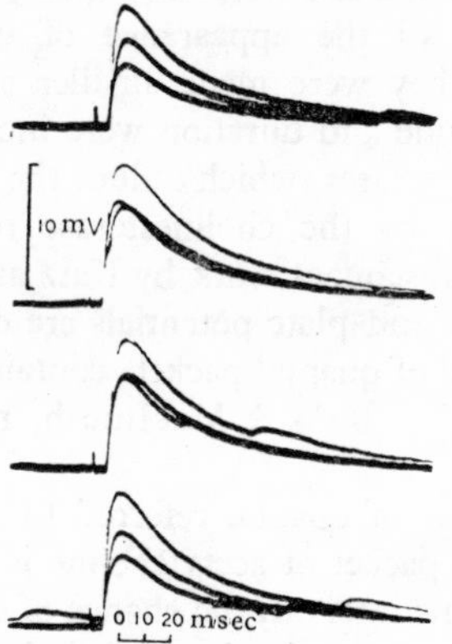

FIG. 9. Fluctuation of e.p.p. response at a single nerve-muscle junction treated with 10 mM-Mg. (Ca concentration was normal: 1·8 mM; prostigmine 10^{-6}.) Intracellular recording. In each record, three superimposed responses are seen. Note scattered spontaneous miniature potentials.

(From Castillo & Katz, 1954, *J. Physiol.*, **124**, 560, Fig. 1.)

In this manner it was shown that ". . . the normal e.p.p., that is the response of a single end-plate to a nerve impulse, is made up of a synchronization of a few hundred miniature e.p.p.s. . . . It is a momentary increase of the frequency—or statistical probability—of an event which occurs spontaneously at a very low rate" (Katz, 1962). It has been shown, in fact, for the cat's tenuissimus muscle that miniature e.p.p.s are about 0·5 mV in size and that the normal end-plate potential is the result of a synchronous release from the nerve terminal of about 200–300 quanta of acetylcholine (Boyd & Martin, 1956). One has therefore to picture acetylcholine as synthesized at the motor nerve terminal and stored there in quanta, perhaps within the synaptic vesicles that can be seen with the electron microscope; the terminal membrane must, however, be leaky, for there is a continual randomly timed escape of quanta under conditions of rest. The arrival of an action potential in the motor terminal produces the synchronous ejection of a number of quanta of the humoral transmitter that is some three times larger than is necessary for transmission from nerve to resting muscle. It is because of this large safety factor in normal neuromuscular transmission that conduction from nerve to muscle is usually a wholly predictable event.

Since it is commonly assumed that transmission between nerve cells in the central nervous system is also humoral, it would be reasonable to expect some evidence of an equivalent synaptic noise in intracellular records from central neurones (Eccles, 1964). Li (1959, 1961) has observed small brief depolarizations of about 0·5 mV when recording from cells in the somato-sensory cerebral cortex of lightly anaesthetized cats. The frequency of these 'spontaneous' random potentials was increased by rubbing the animals' limbs on the experimental table. Artificial stimuli given to the superficial radial nerve could cause a summation of the small potentials which sometimes resulted in a spike discharge. Li concluded ". . . that the small potentials were unitary synaptic potentials or miniature excitatory postsynaptic potentials (miniature e.p.s.p.s) similar to miniature end-plate potentials recorded from neuromuscular junctions". His evidence seems to me in favour of the former hypothesis. If these were really miniature e.p.s.p.s, one would expect the asynchronous excitation of sensory nerves resulting from rubbing the limbs to produce an increase in amplitude rather than an increase in frequency of these signals. Moreover, his observation that their frequency is extremely sensitive to the depth of anaesthesia seems more consistent with their being "unitary synaptic potentials".

In any case, for a number of reasons, one would expect miniature excitatory post-synaptic potentials to be extremely hard to detect in the central nervous system. The size of post-synaptic excitatory potentials recorded with a micropipette in the main body of the cell must depend upon the proximity of these local unitary depolarizations; afferent terminals upon the cell's dendrites would be expected to produce smaller e.p.s.p.s than would those endings upon the soma (Fatt, 1957*a*, *b*; Wall, 1965). Presumably Li's 'unitary snyaptic potential' can be defined as the disturbance of membrane potential set up by one action potential in a single fibre, some of the terminal branches of which make synaptic contact with the cell in question. Unlike the situation obtaining at the neuromuscular junction, central unitary e.p.s.p.s must be far below the threshold for discharge of the neurone, if they are to provide facilities for temporal and spatial summation. Thus, a quantal leakage of 1/100, the amount of transmitter that was normally released by afferent activity (as was found by Katz and Fatt for the neuromuscular junction), would be very hard to detect. Moreover, as we have pointed out already, in the unanaesthetized or lightly anaesthetized animal, many central neurones are continually active. This is likely to provide a randomly timed series of unitary e.p.s.p.s in any cell under observation; a series of signals that would be very difficult to distinguish from the supposed random depolarizations produced by transmitter leakage.

We must conclude that this question remains unanswered. By analogy with the neuromuscular junction, one would expect some spontaneous escape of such humoral transmitters as there may be within the central nervous system. Such leakage would necessarily contribute toward the stochastic behaviour of central neurones, which is further discussed on p. 68. At present, however, there is no convincing evidence that it occurs. In the current state of technical knowledge, it would in fact be a very difficult hypothesis to test.

Probability and sensory neurones

One usually thinks of sensory nerve fibres as supplying the central nervous system with a regular series of action potentials. Illustrations in contemporary textbooks show a regularly spaced series of signals from sensory endings that do not accommodate, while the trains of action potentials set up by the more rapidly accommodating endings display a series of progressively increasing times between neighbouring signals. Where the mean frequency of afferent discharge is not constant, it appears to change according to some law which makes prediction of the exact time of any action potential possible, provided one has information about the times of preceding signals. Nevertheless, it has been shown that there is an element of uncertainty about the timing of a system as simple as the proprioceptive afferents from skeletal muscle.

Hagiwara (1954) examined the trains of afferent discharges set up by a muscle spindle of the frog's sartorius when the muscle was under constant load. He found that the train of signals was not perfectly regular; when the spindle was discharging with a constant mean frequency, there was a random scatter of the time intervals between neighbouring signals about a mean or more probable value. The standard error of these intervals was greater, the lower the mean frequency of discharge. He regarded his results as showing that two independent processes contributed toward the timing of the next action potential in a series. The first of these was considered to be a wholly predictable recovery of threshold T_p of the form:

$$T_p = A \, . \, \text{Exp}\,(c/t)$$

where A was the rheobase of the sensory fibre, t represented the time since the last action potential and c was a constant for the particular afferent. The second contributing factor, he considered to be an unpredictable, relatively small variation in threshold T_u, such that:

$$T_u = f(t) \qquad \text{(some function of } t\text{)}$$

where $f(t)$ "... is a random normal process, the mean being 0 and standard deviation, σ, being a constant", for a given nerve fibre. Thus, when the constant generator potential G (Gray, 1959) produced by a constant load exceeded $(T_p + T_u)$, the next action potential would occur. In this way, the intervals, t, between signals would follow the formula:

$$A \, . \, \text{Exp}\,(c/t) + f(t) = G = \text{Constant}$$

The observed variation of standard deviation of t with change in mean value of t (alteration of mean frequency of discharge) was consistent with this interpretation. Buller, Nicholls & Strom (1953) had also examined the same preparation and recorded small differences in the intervals between consecutive action potentials; although they did not subject the hypothesis to any quantitative test, they suggested that "... superimposed upon the steady level of depolarization there might be small fluctuations of fixed r.m.s. voltage due to thermal agitation of ions, or other causes in the nerve endings, these fluctuations being responsible for the irregularity in impulse irritations". Firth (1966) has provided a similar analysis of interspike intervals for the crayfish stretch receptor.

It is perhaps less surprising that the input from a more complex sensory system such as the retina, should be stochastic in form. Kuffler, Fitzhugh & Barlow (1957) examined afferent discharges from the unanaesthetized eye by recording from single retinal ganglion cells in the decerebrate, unanaesthetized cat. They reported that "... maintained discharges were seen in all ganglion cells during steady illumination of their receptive fields, as well as in complete darkness". Although all ganglion cells showed this steady discharge of action potentials, they did not all respond to illumination in the same way. Altering the steady level of illumination would cause some ganglion cells to increase their rate of discharge to a new maintained frequency; others would respond to the same change by a maintained reduction in firing rate, while the mean frequency of discharge of some units was practically unaffected by this manoeuvre. The short-lasting responses of ganglion cells to changes of illumination within their receptive fields were superimposed upon this steady discharge, so that one might regard visual stimuli as ". . . modulating the ever present background activity" (Kuffler, Fitzhugh & Barlow, 1957).

Although the mean frequency of discharges per minute was steady provided that the illumination of the retina was constant, there was considerable uncertainty about the precise times of firing. The immediate responses to local change of illumination, within the receptive field of a ganglion cell, were superimposed upon this background noise, with the consequence that no two responses to identical stimuli were exactly the same (Fig. 10). Fitzhugh (1957) has attempted an analysis

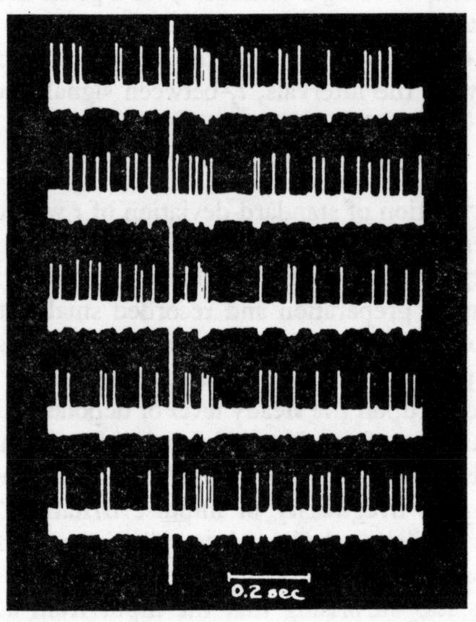

FIG. 10. Photographs of the impulses recorded from an on-centre ganglion cell in response to five successive flashes given at a rate of 1/sec. Flash duration 5 msec; flashes occur at long vertical line. Stimulus intensity 1·74 times threshold. The abscissa is time. Retouched photographs. (From Fitzhugh, 1957, *J. gen. Physiol.*, **40**, 925, Fig. 1.)

of the relation between stimulus and response in these circumstances. This he did by constructing what would now be known as a series of post-stimulus histograms, showing the number of times that the cell fired at various time intervals after the *average* stimulus (Fig. 11). Thus, the abscissa of Fig. 11 shows the time in milliseconds after a 5 msec flash presented within the appropriate receptive field; the ordinate shows the mean numbers of impulses occurring in each 10 msec period subsequent to the stimulus, obtained by averaging the responses to ten

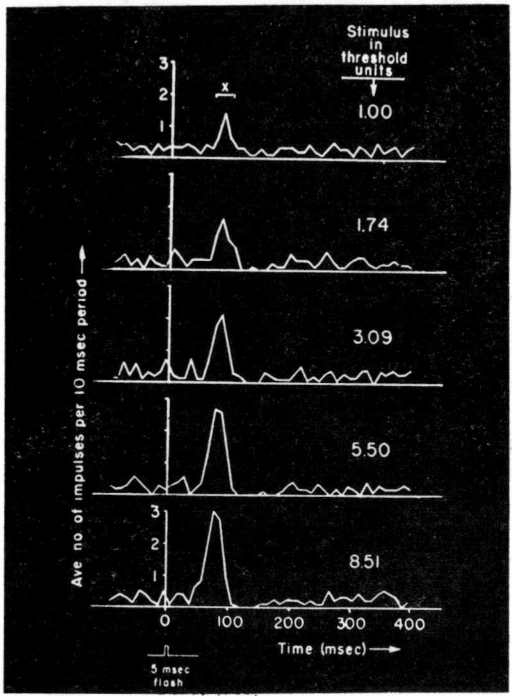

FIG. 11. Transient changes of average frequency following 5 msec flashes, plotted from data such as those of Fig. 10. On the vertical axis is plotted the mean number of impulses in each 10 msec period obtained by averaging over ten successive flashes. The relative stimulus intensity for each curve is as shown, with threshold taken as 1·00. The number of impulses (x) occurring in each discharge during the critical period, marked at the top of the figure, was used as an index of the response.
(From Fitzhugh. 1957, *J. gen. Physiol.*, **40**, 925, Fig. 1.)

consecutive flashes. Plotted in this way, the responses of Fig. 10 are quite easy to see; however, their magnitude cannot be taken as the uncorrected area beneath each 'triangular' response, since this measure would include those action potentials that would have occurred without the presentation of a stimulus. Fitzhugh measured average responses to light flash as the difference between the responses illustrated in Fig. 11 and the computed 'responses' to light flashes of zero intensity (Chapter 3 provides further discussion of the various ways in which responses can be assessed from post-stimulus histograms). Clearly in these circumstances, any statement attempting to relate an individual response to a particular single stimulus, would be senseless. The only meaningful statement that can be made about the relation between stimulus strength and sensory response must be in terms of average behaviour.

Fitzhugh pointed out that the unpredictable nature of retinal responses to weak stimuli necessarily reduced the efficiency of communication between eye and brain. "The problem of analysis of a nerve fibre message by the brain is similar to the engineering problem of detection of a signal in a noisy communication channel." The presence of background noise of the type first reported by Barlow, Fitzhugh & Kuffler must make it harder for the brain 'to decide' when an unexpectedly high frequency of action potentials arrives; harder than it would be if the sensory signal were not contaminated by the presence of spontaneous activity at rest. One must remember, however, that even small light sources will excite many optic nerve fibres simultaneously; during normal activity, a physiologically-meaningful message in the optic nerve trunk will be conveyed by groups of fibres, many of which are doing the same thing at the same time. Fitzhugh (1957) calculated that the threshold for one hundred 'simultaneously excited' ganglion cells should be about 1/20th that for a single unit. The way in which transmission of information increases with increase in the number of simultaneously active channels is discussed at greater length in Chapter 5.

Involuntary eye movements: physiological nystagmus

During voluntary fixation of a visual target, the direction of gaze *appears* to be constant; in fact, sensitive records of eye movement show that this is not so. Both eyes exhibit continual small movements, often referred to as physiological nystagmus, such that their optic axes swing unpredictably in all directions within a small cone of angle which includes the target. Thus, while the most probable direction of gaze can be stated with confidence, the instantaneous orientations of the optic axes are much less certain. These involuntary movements of the eyes are apparently essential to normal perception; the consequent continual movement of images across the retina is a necessary part of normal vision. If some optical device is used to maintain the position of an image constant upon the retina, despite involuntary movements of the eye, perception of simple patterns will fail after some 5 seconds, while the perception of complex patterns becomes distorted by fragmentation.

Although these facts have been known since 1950, they have not yet become a part of accepted physiological literature. At the time of writing, none of five physiological textbooks that I have searched makes any reference to them in the section devoted to the special senses. This information is clearly of vital importance to a proper understanding of the normal or pathologically disturbed visual system, and its omission from these current texts is an unhappy example of the isolation of psychological from neurophysiological literature.

Although the presence of small involuntary movements of the human eye during fixation of a visual target had been described earlier, Ratliff and Riggs provided the first detailed analysis of these movements in 1950. They listed (Ratliff & Riggs, 1950) three types of movement. First, a fine tremor consisting of an irregular movement of high frequency between 30–70 c/s with a median amplitude of some 20 seconds of arc; second, rapid flicks or 'saccades' occurring at irregular intervals averaging about 1/sec., with an amplitude of a few minutes of arc; thirdly, between saccades, they observed slow drifts of unpredictable direction. The high frequency tremor was, as it were, superimposed upon the less frequent changes in the direction caused by drifts and saccades. These results were confirmed by Ditchburn & Ginsborg (1953) who also divided the recorded movements into three categories "... (a) tremor of 10–30″ arc, 30–80 c/s; (b) flicks 1–20′ arc, occupying 0·025 sec; (c) drifts up to 6′ in an interflick period". They described the total movement of the image of a small fixation target relative to the retina as being confined to an area of 100 μ diameter. They suggested, moreover, that the flicks or saccades were responsible for restricting the wandering of the image to this area, since they appeared to provide rapid corrections to the slow drifts, thereby shifting the target's image towards the centre of this area. Figure 12 illustrates the wanderings of a point-target's image across the retina during voluntary fixation; in this case the image was maintained within a circle of diameter equal to about 25 cones. The slow drifts are shown as interrupted lines and have no particular orientation. In contrast, the saccades, shown as continuous lines, are all directed away from the nearest edge of the surrounding circle. The frequency of saccades (and drifts) in this sample is some 2/sec.

It has also proved possible in man to record the movements of both eyes simultaneously. Saccades of one eye seem to be invariably accompanied by saccades in the other eye, which are almost always similar in direction and amplitude. The eye with the greatest error of aim makes the larger saccadic movement and appears to trigger movement of the other eye (Krauskopf, Cornsweet & Riggs, 1960; Riggs & Niehl, 1960).

It is not easy to prevent the movements of physiological nystagmus in man. On the other hand, it is possible to prevent the consequent continual wandering of the image across the retina. One method for producing retinal stabilization of the image, despite small involuntary eye-movements, is to form a visual target from light reflected off a mirror attached to a contact glass carried by the observer's eye. The various optical pathways can be so arranged that any angular movement of the eye carries the target through the same angular arc, with the

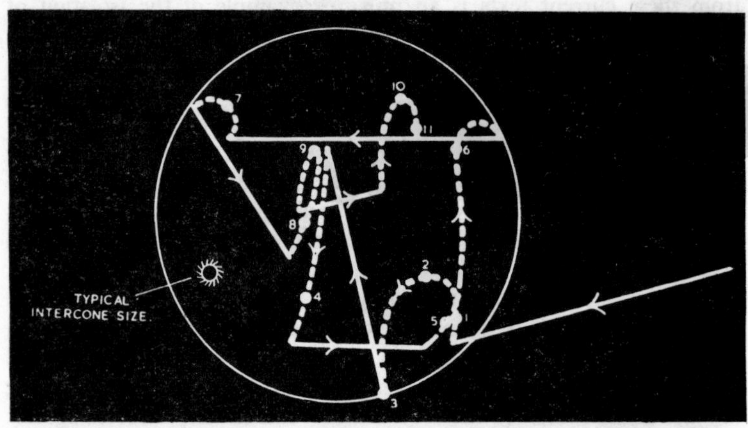

FIG. 12. Movement of the image of a point object on the retina. The large circle is of radius 25 μ (5 min arc); - - - - represents slow drifts; —— represents rapid flicks. Numbered dots indicate order in which movements are made and are spaced at equal time intervals of 200 msec. On this particular occasion the whole movement is within a 25 μ radius circle, but longer period records reveal movements within a circle of radius 50 μ.
(From Ditchburn, 1956, *Problems in Contemporary Optics*, Fig. 5, Arcetri-Firenze: Istituto Nationale di ottica.)

consequence that the target's image remains in one position on the retina (Ditchburn & Fender, 1955). Another technique for the production of stabilized images involves the use of a minute projector which is carried by a contact glass and projects a focused image upon the retina. When the eye moves, so does the contact glass and projector; consequently there is no relative movement between image and retina (Pritchard, 1958). A third method depends upon the production of an after-image by exposing the eye briefly to a very bright target (Bennet-Clark & Evans, 1963). Stabilization of the image by any of these devices causes an observer to report the complete disappearance of simple targets, such as straight light-dark boundaries, after some five seconds or so (Ditchburn & Ginsborg, 1952; Riggs, Ratliff, Cornsweet & Cornsweet, 1953; Yarbus, 1957). The perception of more complex stabilized targets suffers the same sort of rapid decay, but is usually followed by transient reappearance of various component elements of the whole pattern, referred to as fragmentation of the original field (Pritchard, Heron & Hebb, 1960; Bennet-Clark & Evans, 1963). There is considerable argument about the proper interpretation of these partial reappearances (Barlow, 1963), but for our present purposes, it seems more important that the greater part of the stabilized image disappears completely.

There seems no doubt, therefore, that normal vision requires the continual movement of the retinal image that is provided by physiological nystagmus. Ditchburn, Fender & Mayne (1959) tried to find out which of the three components of physiological nystagmus was essential to maintained perception. This they did by imposing controlled movements upon an otherwise stabilized retinal image. They found that "... imposed motion, similar to the drift-component of normal eye movements, has little effect in preventing the 'fade-out' which occurs with a stabilized image. Imposed motion similar to a natural flick produces a sharp regeneration of the image which then fades out again. It is concluded that the flick motion plays a part in maintaining vision but is not the only effect operative in this respect." The saccades themselves seem to be driven by the visual system, for Cornsweet (1956) has found that there are many fewer saccades during stabilized than during normal vision; the rate of drift was the same for both conditions. Cornsweet concludes, "As the retinal image drifts farther and farther away from some particular region of the retina, it becomes more and more likely that a saccadic movement will occur, tending to return the retinal image to that particular region."

The errors of fixation resulting from physiological nystagmus were once regarded as the unwanted consequence of muscle tremor. Skeletal muscles, far larger than the extrinsic muscles of the eye, exhibit tremor of small amplitude when a specified target of pressure or joint flexion is voluntarily maintained (Hammond, Merton & Sutton, 1956). Fluctuations in contraction are cyclical with a dominant frequency of some 10/sec. These variations in activity could be expected from any goal-seeking system (p. 10), and Campbell, Robson & Westheimer (1959) have stressed the similarity between the instability of the finger flexors and that of the ciliary muscle operating the lens, when both are 'holding' steady targets (Fig. 13). Undoubtedly, the alternate movements described above as drifts and saccades belong to the same general class of instability—the hunting errors of a goal-seeking system. The fine 30–80 c/s tremor which is superimposed upon the slower involuntary movements, is probably the result of the small size of eye muscles. The extrinsic eye muscles contain approximately 250 motor units and some 2,000 striated muscle fibres (Torre, 1953). One imagines that the fine tremor of voluntary fixation represents an imperfectly fused tetanic contraction resulting from the periodic discharge of a small number of active motor units. The small size of motor units in the ocular muscle—some 8 muscle fibres per motoneurone as compared with about 150 muscle fibres per unit in the larger limb muscles (Eccles & Sherrington, 1930; Clark, 1931)—probably indicates the effort made by nature to minimize this deficiency.

The instability displayed by most active skeletal muscles, and that

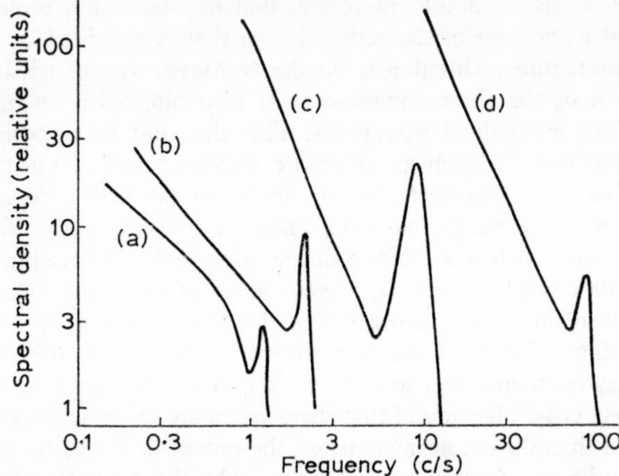

FIG. 13. Frequency spectra of various motor systems in a steady environment, drawn to show principal features (logarithmic coordinates).
(*a*) Pupil diameter during steady illumination of the retina;
(*b*) accommodation during steady viewing of near target;
(*c*) finger displacement during steady pointing;
(*d*) eyeball position during steady fixation (between saccadic movements).
This spectrum was obtained by analysing a record kindly provided by Dr. D. H. Fender.
(From Campbell, Robson & Westheimer, 1959, *J. Physiol.*, **145**, 579, Fig. 12.)

of the ciliary muscle or of the iris, can justly be regarded as the necessary deficiency of a cybernetic system. This generalization would, however, be misleading if applied to the ocular muscles, for without such movements, normal perception would fail. That part of the central nervous system essential to normal perception appears to respond only to local change of retinal illumination. This is somewhat surprising, since it is known that the mammalian optic nerve carries continuous information about the absolute value of local illumination (Kuffler, Fitzhugh & Barlow, 1957). This 'direct-coupled' information must be employed at some lower level within the central nervous system. For instance, it is essential to the control of pupilary aperture.

The observation that stabilized images fragment or disappear, implies that we can best perceive local changes of retinal illumination; that some part of the central nervous system can only respond to the mobile light–dark edges or gradients of intensity within a retinal pattern. (Evidence that this is true for cells of the visual cerebral cortex will be presented in a later chapter.) In fact, there is little loss of knowledge about a patterned field, if the information transmitted reports only the position and magnitude of spatial gradients of light intensity—$\delta I/\delta\theta$, where I = light intensity and θ represents angle of vision. Information about the pattern will be reduced in proportion to $\delta\theta$, the minimum angular displacement over which the nervous system can measure intensity differences. To make this point clearer, Fig. 14 is supposed to represent ten cones

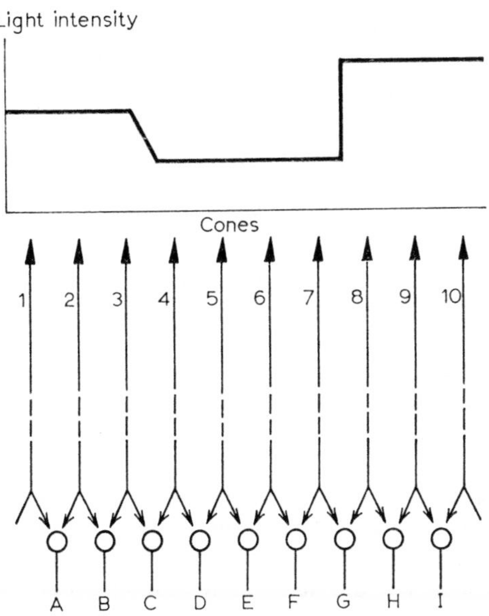

FIG. 14. Illustrating the functional connections of cones (numbered) with cortical units (lettered). (See text.)

in the human fovea, exposed to the indicated distribution of light intensity. The cells at the bottom of the figure represent those neurones within the central nervous system that must record the pattern. Provided the central neurones, C and G, record correctly the difference of intensity between cones 3 and 4, and cones 7 and 8 respectively, the whole pattern can be reconstructed. The resultant reconstruction would not reveal, however, the fact that the gradient of light intensity between cones 3 and 4 was less than that between 7 and 8; in this diagram the separation of cones represents $\delta\theta$ of the preceding argument. Although there is some loss of information in a system which only responds to intensity gradients, there is a considerable economy of activity required to represent the pattern. In the example of Fig. 14, the complete pattern could be recorded by activity of only two central neurones—C and G. If each of the lower row had been connected to one cone, so as to register absolute local intensity, then all nine central neurones would have to be active in order to record the pattern correctly. Thus, by sacrificing a little information, the system of Fig. 14 effects a great economy in active parts.

These considerations show how experiments with human eye movements during fixation and the results of tests with stabilized images provide clear indications of the types of physiological mechanisms likely to be encountered during a neurophysiological investigation of central visual processes. Assuming the visual cerebral cortex to be essential to perception, one would expect to find that neurones there were little affected by continuous, stationary retinal illumination; their function would be to indicate local changes of light intensity. Moreover, one might expect the cortex to be built on the principle that the smallest possible number of visual units should be activated by the retinae at any one time. To a large extent these expectations have been justified by recent neurophysiological results, but a full discussion of these will be deferred until Chapter 5.

Physiological nystagmus has been dealt with here at some length, since it exemplifies a 'peripheral' system whose stochastic nature is essential to normal function. It is true that we might see as well if involuntary eye movements were cyclical and wholly predictable in direction and frequency. However, it appears that the mammalian visual system has 'made good use' of a deficiency, inherent to the necessary tracking mechanism. As it is, the signals to which the neurones of the central nervous system must respond during voluntary fixation are, to some extent, both spatially and temporally unpredictable. Cells of visual cortex, for instance, can only indicate the temporal and spatial average of the afferent signals they receive.

CHAPTER 3

METHODS OF STATISTICAL ANALYSIS

RECORDS FROM LARGE ELECTRODES

Average evoked responses

The development of averaging techniques for neurophysiology began with attempts to record with large electrodes the responses of intact and continually active brain, evoked by sensory stimulation. Since Dawson's first success in this field, the popularity of computers in neurophysiology has steadily increased as the power of these new analytic methods became apparent.

One of the earliest and simplest techniques employed for extracting an evoked response from the random background of spontaneous activity was the use of superimposed photographs (Dawson, 1947, 1950). The electroencephalogram or electrocorticogram, recorded with gross electrodes, is displayed upon an oscilloscope screen; the sweep of the oscilloscope is triggered at the time of each sensory stimulus. The shutter of a camera is held open during a period of stimulation so that a photograph is obtained of several sweeps superimposed. A record of this sort is shown in Fig. 6. Such records show up the *most common* voltage changes that follow the average stimulus as a trace which is denser and broader than that left by the less common changes. The time course of this most common voltage is not, of course, the same as the time course of *mean* voltage following the average stimulus. Moreover, the superimposed record cannot easily be described in numerical terms, since its form depends upon the width of the oscilloscope trace and the light/density curve of the photographic emulsion that is used. Nevertheless, the method can prove extremely useful for qualitative work in circumstances where similar responses occasionally follow identical stimuli, as is often the case with the anaesthetized brain. The technique is not much use where the level of spontaneous activity is so high that the oscilloscope traces rarely follow similar paths; in this situation a true averaging procedure is far more informative.

In 1951, Dawson published a note describing briefly an automatic method for obtaining the mean potential at various times after the average stimulus; his method was later described in detail (Dawson, 1951, 1954). Sensory stimuli were given at a steady frequency and in the interval between consecutive stimuli, a single-pole, many-way switch rotated exactly once; if the switch is visualized as having N

equally spaced contacts, then the duration of contact between wiper and any one contact would be a little less than I/N, where I = the time interval between stimuli. Thus, the time between stimuli was divided into N equal segments of δT. The voltage from the output of the recording amplifier was fed to the wiper of the rotating switch; in this way, the potential recorded between $(n-1)\delta T$ and $n \,.\, \delta T$ after every stimulus was fed to the *nth* contact of the switch. A condenser attached to each contact of the rotating switch operated as a storage 'bin' and accumulated a charge proportional to the sum of all the voltages that had been briefly applied to the relevant contact. Fig. 15 is taken from Dawson's original paper.

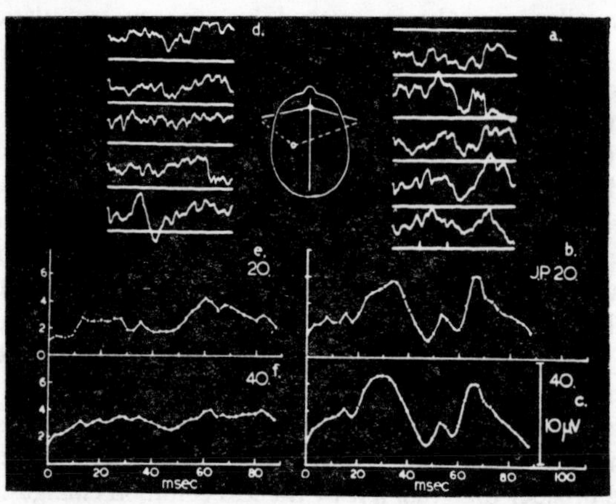

FIG. 15. A sample of 5 records from a set of 40, with the stimulus applied to the right arm and the record from the left scalp, is shown in (*a*). In these records the responses are not clear amongst the spontaneous activity. The averages of 20 and 40 records are shown in (*b*) and (*c*). Control records in (*d*), with no stimulus applied, show averages like (*e*) and (*f*). The stimuli were applied at the times of the dots below the traces and the marks on the lowest trace in (*a*) show an interval of 20 msec. The calibration to the right of (*c*) shows the deflection due to 10 μV.

(From Dawson, 1954, *Electroen. Neurophysiol.*, **6,** 65.)

The mechanical nature of Dawson's instrument presented certain disadvantages; it necessitated, for instance, an inflexible timing of stimulation and, consequently, randomly timed stimuli could not be used. However, the sorting of potentials and their allocations into appropriate time bins can be performed electronically and many instruments have since been designed that do exactly the same job without the use of moving parts (Brazier & Casby, 1952; Barlow, 1957; Smith & Burns, 1960; Burns, Ferch & Mandl, 1965). Some of these instruments can also be employed to calculate the average cross-correlation between records obtained from two independent gross electrodes, or will provide the autocorrelation of a record from one electrode (Brazier, 1961).

Interpretation of gross responses

The post-stimulus histogram computed by Dawson's machine, or by any of the later variants, provides for various times after the average stimulus a statement of the mean potential recorded with a large electrode at a considerable distance from the source of voltage. The source is usually the simultaneous activity of many nerve cells and, for this reason, the large electrode is continually recording a kind of spatial average related to the behaviour of a large population of units. Brazier (1949, 1961) provides a formula for calculating the distribution of potential across the surface of a conducting sphere when a radially oriented dipole is active within the sphere (Fig. 16). Although this distribution is not exponential, one might speak about the space constant of potential gradient, as the distance from the focal point at which the potential has fallen to $1/e$ (or approximately 1/3) of its maximum value. In the case of e.e.g. recordings from the scalp, with a dipole in the cerebral cortex 3 cm below, the space constant would be about 2 cm. For gross electrodes resting directly upon the cerebral cortex, the effective space constant for a dipole 1 mm below the cortical surface would be some 2 mm. One is reminded of Adrian and Matthews' statement (1934), "In the anaesthetized, but uninjured, brain the neurones tend to pulsate in small groups covering an area not more than 3–4 mm diameter. Periodic waves of activity may spread over the whole cortex in deep anaesthesia, but the neurones which take part in it still react in small groups which pulsate out of phase with one another." The cerebral cortex lying beneath a surface-circle of 2 mm radius contains approximately half a million cell bodies. It appears, therefore, that the record from a gross electrode on the cortical surface must be significantly influenced by the activity of a very large number of neurones. The resultant record cannot usefully be regarded as a spatial average, since the contribution of each active neurone to the potential record will depend upon its distance, its orientation and its physiological class. One knows, for instance, that central neurones belonging to quite different functional categories often lie next to one another; in the brain stem, the same micropipette often records the alternate bursts of activity of both inspiratory and expiratory neurones (Salmoiraghi & Burns, 1960).

For these reasons, recordings from gross electrodes are often hard or impossible to interpret. The summation of many gross responses that is needed for the production of a P.S.H. or average evoked response in no way removes these difficulties. Thus, while the procedure of temporal

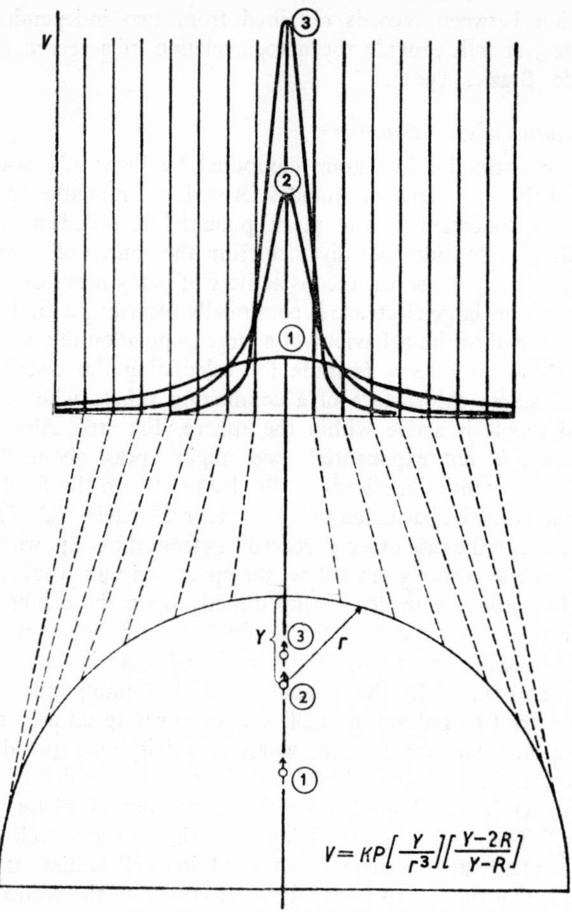

FIG. 16. Voltage as the function of recording position on surface of a sphere for 3 positions of a dipole. Voltage distribution on surface of a sphere caused by dipoles at various depths below the surface. *Y*, distance of dipole from surface on the radius, *R*, of sphere; *r*, distance of recording electrode from dipole; *K*, constant; *P*, dipole moment (4).
(From Brazier, 1961, *Meth. med. Res.*, **9,** 405, Fig. 15.)

averaging has been of great use in the clinical field, as a tool for the localization of malfunction, it has provided little new understanding of neural mechanisms.

THE ANALYSIS OF DIGITAL RECORDS

Averaging procedures that are essentially similar may be applied to the records of unit activity obtained with micro-electrodes. In this case, however, the signal of activity is usually digital (all-or-nothing) in nature and consequently it is not the magnitude of the signal but the time of firing which is of interest. The relatively long records needed for the determination of average behaviour are most readily obtained from extracellular micro-electrodes which, unlike the intracellular micropipette, are easily maintained within recording distance of one unit for periods of an hour or more. Nevertheless, the production of records suitable for statistical analysis presents certain problems that are not associated with the use of larger recording electrodes. In order to maintain a satisfactory signal-to-noise ratio, it is necessary to keep the tip of the extracellular electrode within some 15 μ of the soma wall (Svaetichin, 1951; Mountcastle, Davies & Berman, 1957; Burns, 1961), and such proximity of a foreign body is only tolerated by the recorded unit provided there is virtually no relative movement of electrode and cell. Various devices have been employed to reduce relative movement to a minimum. The two most successful methods are probably the closed-skull technique and the 'floating' micro-electrode (Burns, 1961). The first of these reduces the expansion and contraction of brain volume which accompany respiration and the heart beat by maintaining a closed and water-filled cranial cavity; the second method permits work with the exposed brain by suspending the micro-electrode from a very weak spring so that the electrode follows the relatively slow movements of the brain (Burns & Robson, 1960). Despite these precautions, it is important to remember that the slight mechanical disturbance caused by cautious approach to a cell, or that caused by readjustment of an electrode while recording, may be sufficient to make a temporary change in the behaviour of the unit. Many spontaneously-active units fire less often soon after the arrival of the micro-electrode's tip in their vicinity, but recover a steady discharge rate some two or three minutes after the electrode becomes stationary; a transient depression of firing rate also sometimes accompanies readjustment of electrode position. Cells often recover stable behaviour a few minutes after the well-known injury discharge caused by collision of the exploring electrode with some part of the unit's membrane. These changes in discharge frequency that can accompany electrode movement clearly indicate a transient alteration of excitability to all incoming stimuli, for they are always accompanied by similar changes in response to test stimuli. Thus a cell in the visual cortex which is slightly injured by electrode movement will show a short-lasting increase in mean frequency accompanied by a transient increase in responsiveness to retinal excitation.

In general, this sensitivity of units to the recording electrode demands a degree of care in the preparation of records for statistical analysis that is unnecessary with larger electrodes.

Slow movements of the electrode relative to the recorded unit do not appear to alter the cells' behaviour in any way, but they can cause considerable changes in the size of the recorded signals. Thus, over a period of an hour there is commonly some drift in the magnitude of action potentials that undoubtedly originated from the same unit throughout. Even when there is no electrode movement, action potentials from one unit do not usually present as a series of spikes of identical height. This is because they are often recorded at relatively high gain and consequently appear superimposed upon a background of considerable noise. One becomes suspicious that the micro-electrode is picking up signals from more than one unit if the variation in height of neighbouring action potentials exceeds the amplitude of base-line noise. Clearly, it is theoretically possible for the electrode to be so placed that the signals from two nearby cells are indistinguishable, and very occasionally this does occur. The dual nature of the resulting record can usually be identified by making a slight movement of the micro-electrode, which splits the record into two series of spikes of slightly different magnitudes. In all cases of doubt it is wise to submit the record to interval analysis (p. 50); if it contains any intervals between consecutive signals that are less than 1 msec, it probably represents the discharges of more than one cell. Single cortical units discharging spontaneously in the isolated unanaesthetized forebrain rarely show a functional refractory period that is less than 1 msec, although even units with mean frequencies as low as 1 or 2/sec can occasionally fire twice within this time.

Voltage gates

The small variations in signal amplitude, referred to above, make the use of a voltage gate desirable for accurate analysis of the record. In effect, a voltage gate 'draws a horizontal line' along the continuous record of activity and counts any signal that exceeds a chosen size by emitting a standard pulse (Fig. 17). Such an instrument is useful for two reasons. First, it converts the signals on the original record into pulses suitable to the input of any automatic computer that may be employed to scan the record, on-line or at some later time (Burns, Mandl & Smith, 1963; Burns, Ferch & Mandl, 1965). Second, it provides a noise-free auditory signal, which can be extremely helpful during the progress of an experiment. For the latter purpose, however, it is more useful to have an auditory signal whose amplitude varies with the amount by which the original action potential exceeds the pre-set critical voltage (Fig. 17); this makes it possible to judge by ear any

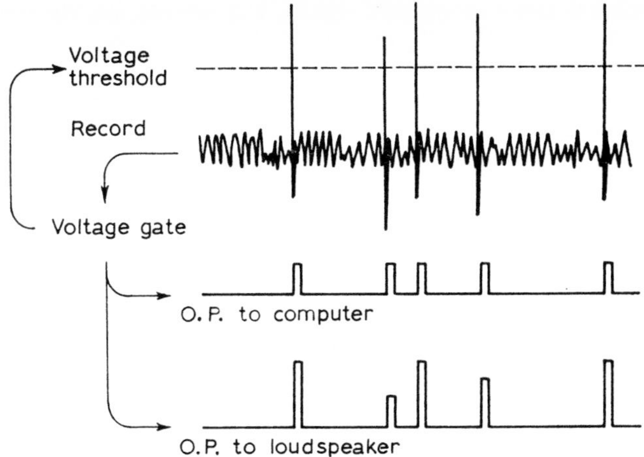

FIG. 17. Illustrating the function of a voltage gate.

change that there may be in the size of the recorded spikes and thus may provide warning that the position of the micro-electrode needs readjustment.

A more complicated, but extremely useful form of voltage gate, is a pulse-height discriminator (Plumb, 1965). An extracellular micro-electrode is often placed so that it records clearly a simultaneous record of the action potentials from two cells, one of which produces larger signals than does the other. A pulse-height discriminator will emit two

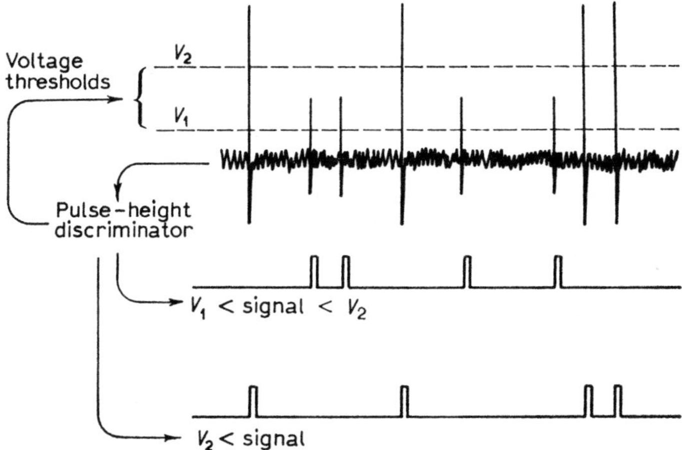

FIG. 18. Use of a pulse-height discriminator for analysing the activities of two cells, recorded with one extracellular micro-electrode.

independent trains of standard signals, one representing the times of firing of the 'smaller cell', the other indicating the behaviour of the 'larger cell' (Fig. 18). In this way, one record can be used to calculate the responses of two neighbouring cells to the same stimulus; a pulse-height discriminator can also be used to form a cross-correlation of the behaviour of two such units.

Mean frequency

There is a large number of ways in which a series of action potentials providing a train of digital signals could transmit information of physiological significance. It does not follow, of course, that the nervous system makes use of all the 'information' carried by an axon that would be classified as such by the communication engineer. In fact, one of the most important questions facing neurophysiologists at present is, "Which aspects of the digital behaviour of central neurones are physiologically meaningful, in that they determine the behaviour of other cells?" Unfortunately, one is not yet in a position to answer this question and a variety of statistical analyses have recently been tried in an empirical attempt to define the critical parameters of neuronal behaviour. The remainder of this chapter is largely devoted to a discussion of some of the methods of analysis that have been explored.

Present evidence suggests that the mean number of discharges per minute of cortical neurones is a relatively unimportant aspect of their behaviour. Many cells in the visual cortex, for instance, display a marked response to retinal excitation, without any change in their mean rate of firing; the action potentials that would have occurred during spontaneous activity in the unstimulated brain are simply redistributed in time (Burns, Heron & Pritchard, 1962). Even when excitation of cortical cells does alter their mean frequency, this measure of their activity invariably seems less sensitive than other parameters of behaviour. Nevertheless, mean frequency is easy to measure and has proved a valuable guide to the elementary properties of central neurones. The responses of central units to the local application of various drugs are usually recorded as alterations of mean discharge rates (Salmoiraghi & Steiner, 1963; Bradley & Wolstencroft, 1964; Krnjevic, 1965). The responses of cortical neurones to both polarization and trans-synaptic excitation have also been recorded in terms of mean frequency per minute (Burns, 1957; Burns, Heron & Pritchard, 1962; Bindman, Lippold & Redfearn, 1964).

Frequency meters for physiological work fall into two categories (Burns, 1961). The simplest form depends upon the charge of a condenser with a fixed leak, by standard pulses of current, each of which is triggered by a voltage gate of the type described above. The rate of charge depends upon the frequency of input; the rate of discharge is proportional to the instantaneous voltage. For a steady input frequency, f, the mean potential, V, across the condenser, C, is given by:

$$\frac{V}{r}=\frac{i\,.\,\delta t\,.\,f}{C} \qquad \text{(Fig. 19)}$$

where i = the current during the charge pulse
δt = the time for which this current flows
r = the leak resistance

from which $V \propto f$.

This form of frequency meter is only suitable for the measurement of frequencies that change slowly relative to RC (the time constant of leakage) and change little by comparison with $1/RC$. Figure 19 illus-

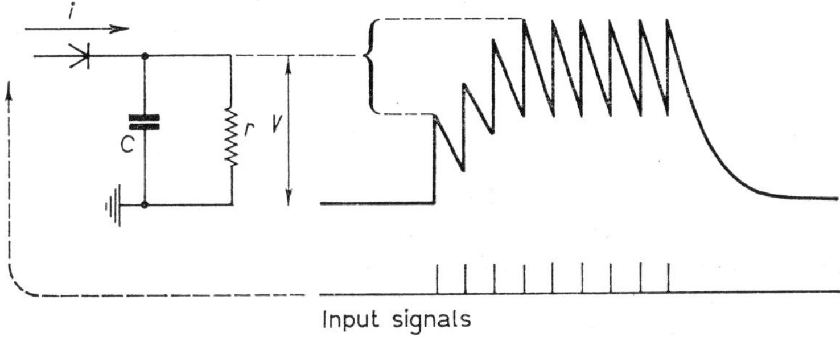

FIG. 19. Illustrating the operation of an RC frequency meter.

trates the way in which a resistance-capacity or RC frequency meter responds to sudden changes of input frequency. The new steady voltage associated with a sudden change of input frequency is approached with a time constant RC. Thus, the useful range of such an instrument is limited by the choice of RC; if RC is too large, the recorder becomes sluggish in response; if RC is too small, the fluctuations of condenser potential about the mean value, V, become inconveniently large.

A much more flexible and accurate frequency meter is provided by any instrument which records the number of events, n, occurring within consecutive identical time intervals, which can be adjusted to any convenient value, T. Many commercially available scalers are admirably suited for this purpose. Alternatively, a less expensive instrument with similar properties can be constructed by allowing brief pulses of constant current to charge up a condenser with virtually no leak. The charge of the condenser is proportional to the number of input signals that have occurred and may be read out through a cathode follower; every T seconds, a switch discharges the condenser, thereby cyclically resetting the count to zero (Burns, Ferch & Mandl, 1965). The response time of such an instrument is given by T, the preset integration period; that is to say, a step change in input frequency will be correctly registered by the output in a time which is not greater than T. More important is the fact that the choice of T does not affect either the sensitivity or the operating range of the recorder.

The value of measurements of the mean firing rate of cells in the cerebral cortex is discussed in Chapters 5 and 6.

Cross-correlation and the post-stimulus histogram

A post-stimulus histogram, or P.S.H., is a cross-correlation between a series of identical stimuli applied to some part of the nervous system and some measure of neural behaviour. As such, it provides a statement about the average response to a series of stimuli. Records of the type first described by Dawson (and discussed above) show the average voltage appearing in the electroencephalogram at various times after a series of identical peripheral stimuli. A similar statistic can be derived from records of unit discharge during test stimulation of the nervous system; in this case, however, it is the average number of spikes occurring at various times after the standard stimuli which is computed. An example of a post-stimulus histogram of this sort has already been given in Fig. 11, taken from Fitzhugh's work. The P.S.H. provides a graph showing the cross-correlation between the times of test stimulation and the times of unit discharge; the abscissa shows time after stimulation, while the ordinate displays the total count of action potentials that occurred between T and $(T+\delta T)$ after stimulation. It provides, of course, the best estimate that can be made of probability that future stimuli of the same sort will be followed by action potentials. Provided that the original record of spike discharges form a stationary series—one in which there is no significant drift of behaviour with time—the accuracy of this estimate will increase with increase in length of record considered. Accuracy will decrease with decrease in the value of δT for the same reason, since the reliability of any predicted count between T and $(T+\delta T)$ depends upon the number of signals falling within this 'time bin' and the number of trials or stimuli used in computing the average count. These points are illustrated in Fig. 20 which shows post-stimulus histograms calculated for a neurone in the visual cerebral cortex during excitation of the retina with a cyclically moving pattern. Figures 20*a* and *b* show how sampling error is reduced by increasing the length of 'stationary' record analysed; they illustrate a rather obvious point. While one should clearly compute the P.S.H. from the longest possible record, there is no such simple rule in the choice of δT. If there were a normal distribution of individual samples about the mean count, n, in a time bin, the standard error of the mean would vary linearly with $1/\delta T$. On the other hand, the error attached to estimation of latency, L, of some identifiable feature of the response, such as the peak counts of Figs. 20*b* and *c*, is proportional to δT. Thus the choice of an optimal value for δT will depend upon the sort of information required. The best value for latency measurements can only be chosen empirically; when δT is too small, some features of the response become masked by the increase in sampling error as illustrated in Fig. 20*c*.

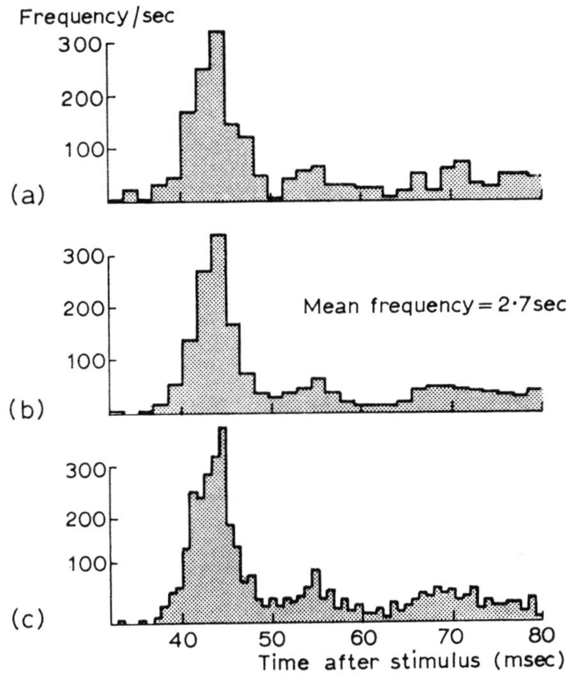

FIG. 20. Three post-stimulus histograms derived from the same record. They show the average response of a neurone in the visual cortex to small, sudden, identical movements of a retinal pattern at time zero.

(*a*) Analysis of 25 seconds of record showing average response to 75 stimuli; $\delta T = 1{\cdot}6$ msec.

(*b*) Analysis of 100 seconds of record showing average response to 300 stimuli; $\delta T = 1{\cdot}6$ msec.

(*c*) The same as (*b*) but analysed with $\delta T = 0{\cdot}8$ msec.

The choice of useful units for the ordinate scale of a post-stimulus histogram presents some difficulty. Ordinate values can be expressed in terms of:

$$\text{Frequency per second} = \frac{(\text{Count in each time bin of } \delta T \text{ duration})}{(\text{Number of stimuli}) \times (\delta T \text{ in seconds})}$$

In this case the P.S.H. would be intended to display the instantaneous frequency of unit firing at various times after the average stimulus. In fact, this is often a legitimate interpretation of the P.S.H., because the latency of any visible peak response is usually the mean of a considerable scatter of individual latencies. But the use of frequency/second for the ordinate can be very misleading when a unit responds, perhaps, to only occasional stimuli, but does so with constant latency. In this case, the count recorded in the time bin collecting the peak score will be the same whatever the value of δT chosen for analysis of the record. Consequently, the estimated frequency/second will appear to be five times higher for $\delta T=1$ msec, than it will when δT is chosen to be 5 msec. It is for this reason that it is sometimes preferable to express P.S.H. ordinates in terms of:

$$\text{Count per stimulus} = \frac{(\text{Count in each bin of } \delta T \text{ duration})}{(\text{Number of stimuli})}$$

while specifying the value of δT chosen for analysis.

The post-stimulus histogram provides a graphical illustration of the *a postiori* probability that a neurone will fire at various times after stimulation. Its form is often complex and can contain several peaks. The presence of two peaks does not necessarily indicate that the unit responded twice to the average stimulus. A neurone which responds only once to each test stimulus, after one of two possible latencies, *l* and *L*, can produce exactly the same P.S.H. as one which sometimes fires twice after a single stimulus. These differences of behaviour can only be separated by exposing the same record to another form of analysis—autocorrelation (see below). This will answer the following question: "In what fraction of trials did the unit discharge twice with consecutive latencies of *l* and *L*?"

It is sometimes convenient to describe the 'response' displayed in the post-stimulus histogram by a single number, so that one may, for instance, state a relation between response and stimulus strength. Choosing an aspect of the P.S.H. to represent the response is not easy; there are many parameters of the P.S.H. which might be selected and unfortunately we do not yet know which properties of central neurones are relevant to the transmission of physiologically meaningful information. Fitzhugh (1957), whose data are quoted (Figs. 10 and 11), measured response as the net difference in behaviours of the stimulated and unstimulated unit; in fact, his measure of response involved subtracting the P.S.H. obtained with zero stimulus strength from that obtained with an effective stimulus. This simple procedure can only be used when it is known that effective stimulation does not alter the overall mean frequency of unit discharge.

Whatever the effect of stimulation upon mean frequency, stimuli that did not influence the temporal distribution of recorded spikes, would by definition yield a P.S.H. in which the expected count, e, in every time bin would be the same. The best estimate of e is given by:

$$e = \frac{S \, . \, N \, . \, \delta T}{T}$$

where N = the number of spikes contributing to the P.S.H.
T = the duration of record analysed
δT = the duration of the time bins used
S = the number of stimuli employed in computing the average response.

Thus, response to the average stimulus can be expressed as some function of $(n-e)$, where n represents the count in each bin. Fitzhugh used $\Sigma(n-e)$ as a measure of response, which is possible with post-stimulus histograms of the form illustrated in Fig. 11; usually, however, the P.S.H. is biphasic or multiphasic and some more complex estimation of net deviation from zero-correlation is required. Burns & Smith (1962) made use of χ^2/e as an objective measure of response, R, so that:

$$R = \frac{\chi^2}{e} = \sum \left\{ \frac{(n-e)^2}{e^2} \right\}$$

One merit of defining response in this way is that the statistical significance of results may be easily calculated. On the other hand, this measure completely disregards the shape of the post-stimulus histograms which it summarizes. Consequently, a weak response can easily be confused with random deviations from the expected mean count, e. In other situations, response has been equated to some simple measure such as:

$$R = \frac{p-e}{e}$$

where p represents the peak count recorded in any time bin (Burns, Heron & Pritchard, 1962). The truth of the matter is that one does not know at present which aspect of the P.S.H. carries essential, physiological information. The problem can only be solved empirically.

It is important to remember that a post-stimulus histogram contains information that is not available to the central nervous system. The experimental animal has no way of knowing when a stimulus occurs other than by reference to the disturbance of neuronal activity which is evoked. Thus while the experimenter can easily perform the cross-correlation that leads to a P.S.H., the nervous system of the experimental animal could never affect a similar computation. The importance of this point is well illustrated by reference to an aspect of the behaviour of units in the cat's visual cerebral cortex (Burns & Pritchard, 1964). When the retina is excited by a simple pattern of light and darkness, to which is given a rectangular cyclical movement, the most stimulating direction of pattern movement for many cortical neurones is determined by whether the unit is representing the relatively light or dark sides of the neighbouring border (Fig. 21). This behaviour on the part of many

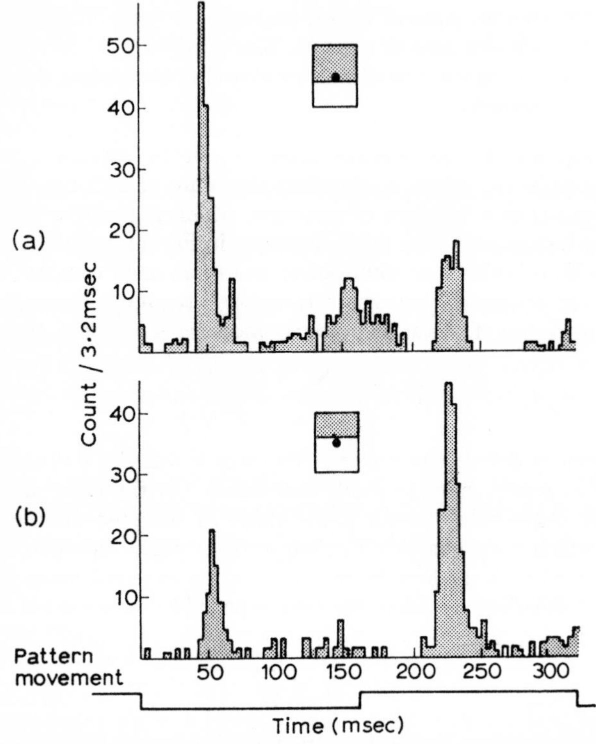

FIG. 21. Post-stimulus histograms from a visual neurone excited by an oscillating, straight black–white border. In (*a*) the representative district for the unit lay 0·5° on the dark side of the border. In (*b*) the same point was 0·5° on the light side of the border.
(From Burns & Pritchard, 1964, *J. Physiol.*, **175**, 445, Fig. 3.)

visual neurones might be considered sufficient to indicate to the rest of the nervous system whether these units were representing the light or dark parts of the visual field, until it is realized that, to use such information for contrast discrimination, the nervous system must be simultaneously informed about the directions of pattern movement. Stated in another way, the nervous system could use this property of visual neurones for contrast discrimination, provided that the output of these units could be correlated with information concerning the directions of the saccadic movements responsible for retinal excitation. The evidence at present available suggests that the necessary information about eye movements is not fed back to higher levels within the central nervous system (Brindley & Merton, 1960).

Although the post-stimulus histogram does not provide a description of information that is available to the central nervous system, it does offer an invaluable analytic tool. It can reveal the presence and magnitude of responses, when these are superimposed upon a noisy background. It describes a number of meaningful and quantitative statements that can be made about the relation between stimulus and response in a stochastic system. Moreover, it offers records from which the latency and refractory period of selected components in the response may be assessed.

The test stimuli used to derive a post-stimulus histogram are usually given at regular intervals, of sufficient length that the response to one stimulus is complete before the next stimulus is provided. The P.S.H. should, therefore, be regarded as a special case of cross-correlation in which the signals of one series occur at regular intervals. This is simply a matter of physiological convenience, for the same sort of analysis can just as readily be applied to two series of irregular events. Thus the same analytic procedure can be used to cross-correlate the times of discharge of two single neurones. The resulting analysis provides estimates of the probabilities that the average discharge of neurone *A* will be followed by a discharge of unit *B* after various intervals of time. The cross-correlogram of Fig. 22 was computed from a record obtained with a single micropipette; the record showed two series of action potentials of different sizes which must have come from two cells separated by some 30 μ within the cat's visual cerebral cortex. It will be seen that cell *A* was very likely to fire some 2 msec after the average discharge of *B*; on the other hand, a discharge of *B* was much less likely to follow the average discharge of unit *A*. Absence of cross-correlation would have provided an essentially horizontal line in these cross-correlograms, and there would have been no statistically significant difference between the counts of the various time bins. It would be obtained if there were no relation between the times of firing of the two units and the two series of signals were strictly independent. The results of Fig. 22 show clearly that the times of discharge of these two cells were not independent. The fact that the discharge of *B* is frequently followed by discharge of *A* indicates either that some common factor was modulating their excitabilities, such as a common source of excitation, or that neurone *B* was frequently responsible for exciting neurone *A*.

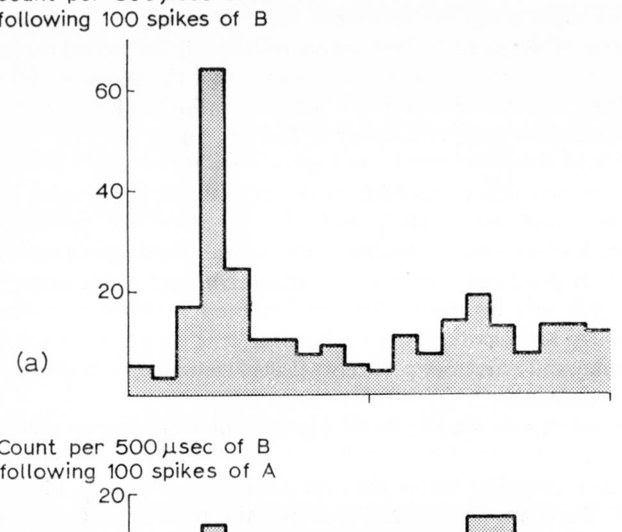

FIG. 22. Cross-correlograms of the spontaneous activity of two neighbouring neurones (*A* and *B*) recorded with one micro-electrode in the parietal cortex of the cat's isolated, unanaesthetized fore-brain.

(*a*) The probability that a discharge of neurone *A* will follow a discharge of unit *B* (at time zero).

(*b*) The probability that discharge of *B* will follow that of *A*.

The problems of summarizing a cross-correlogram in some single measurement which indicates the degree of cross-correlation are those of summarizing response as described by a post-stimulus histogram. As before, some function of $(n-e)$ must be used—some measure of the deviation from the horizontal straight line which would indicate independence of the two functions.

Interval analysis

A graph of interval distribution shows the frequencies with which various intervals between consecutive action potentials have occurred. Figure 23 shows the result of analysing a 214 second record of 2000 spikes from a single neurone in the cat's parietal cortex. The abscissa of this figure shows time since the last discharge in milliseconds; the ordinate indicates the number of intervals between consecutive signals that lay between T and $(T+\delta T)$. It will be seen that there were no intervals less than 1·5 msec, indicating what might be called a *functional refractory period* of this duration; it is also clear from the figure that the most common interval was around 3 msec. We have already pointed out that the functional refractory period of cortical neurones operating under physiological conditions in the isolated, unanaesthetized forebrain is never less than 1 msec and is usually near to this value, whatever the mean frequency or discharge. On the other hand, the position of the peak in the interval distribution curve varies considerably from cell to cell. The ascent of the curve from the origin to this peak presumably provides some indication of the average rate of recovery of excitability of a unit from each previous discharge.

If this cell were firing at random with respect to time, in the sense that it was equally likely to fire within any short period of time δT, then the ordinates of an interval distribution (such as that of Fig. 23*a*) would be given by:

$$n = \frac{N \,.\, \delta T}{I \,.\, \exp\left(-T/I\right)}$$

(Feller, 1950; Fatt & Katz, 1952; Martin & Branch, 1958)

where N = the total number of intervals measured
I = the mean interval between consecutive signals.

The deviations of the actual interval distribution from this prediction (Fig. 23*b*) would be a strict measure of the time-course of excitability, provided that the afferent excitation to the recorded cell were known to be random with respect to time. This is unlikely to be the case, particularly if there is any feed-back from the cell to itself, and one can only refer to such deviations as a *functional recovery curve*, indicating that recovery of excitability contributes something to its shape. The functional recovery curve for the neurone of Fig. 23*a* is plotted in Fig. 23*b*.

Interval distributions have been used to describe the behaviour of peripheral sensory nerves by Buller, Nichols & Strom (1953) and by Hagiwara (1954). They have been used as a test for randomness or unpredictability of firing time for miniature end-plate potentials (Fatt & Katz, 1952), for spinal interneurones by Hunt & Kuno (1959), for spontaneously active Betz cells in the cerebral cortex (Martin & Branch, 1958), and other cortical neurones (Smith & Smith, 1965). Gerstein & Kiang (1960; see also Rodieck, Kiang & Gerstein, 1962), have used interval distributions in the classification of sensory responses among neurones of the cochlear nucleus and the auditory cerebral cortex.

The main value of the interval distribution lies in the information it provides concerning randomness of behaviour and recovery of excitability. Unlike the post-stimulus histogram, an interval distribution

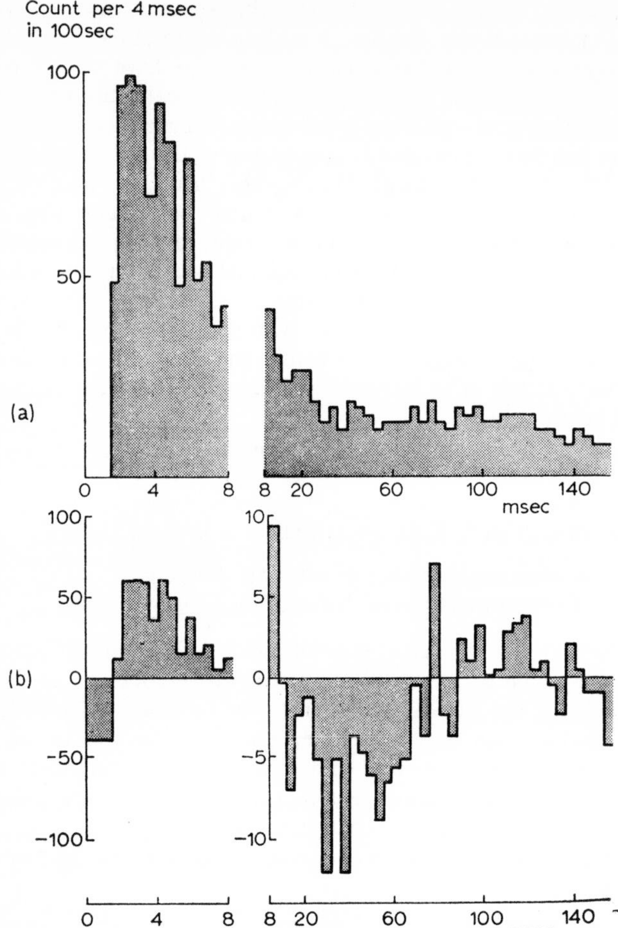

FIG. 23. Interval distributions for a cell in the parietal cortex of a cat's unanaesthetized, isolated forebrain. Spontaneous activity.

(*a*) The distribution of intervals between consecutive spikes in a 214 sec record; mean frequency = 9·36/sec. Note the functional refractory period.

(*b*) The same results plotted as deviations from a Poisson distribution of the same mean frequency; plotted using two different ordinate scales.

describes information, all of which is available to the nervous system of the experimental animal. Moreover, it is information which a Sherringtonian nerve cell could easily use; a neurone which suddenly began to bombard its neighbour with a train of signals displaying a new and shorter most-common interval, becomes more likely to excite that neighbour by virtue of temporal summation. The sensitivity of the interval distribution of cortical neurones to particular forms of visual input will be discussed in Chapter 5.

Autocorrelation

Interval analysis provides the distribution of time intervals between *consecutive* signals in a record of spike discharges (Fig. 24*b*). In contrast,

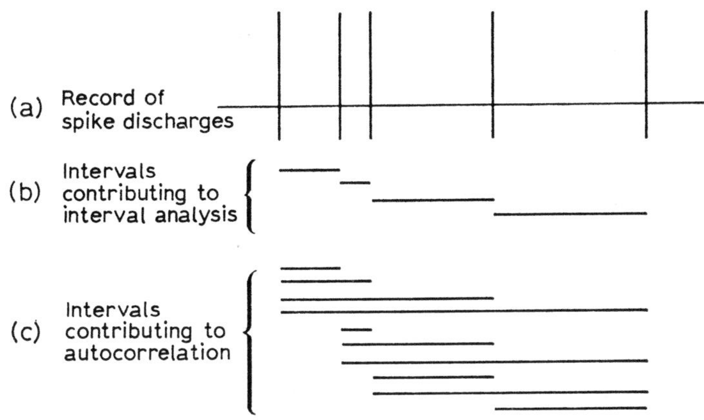

FIG. 24. Illustrating the time intervals contributing to interval analysis and autocorrelations.

the autocorrelogram from a similar record shows the numbers of action potentials which have occurred between T and $(T+\delta T)$ after *any* preceding signal. The process of autocorrelation, therefore, consists in measuring all time intervals of the sort illustrated in Fig. 24*c* and allocating each interval to one of a series of time bins. An interval which was more than $(n-1)\delta T$ and less than $n \, . \, \delta T$ would contribute unity to the total count accumulated in the nth time bin.

The autocorrelogram indicates any tendency toward cyclical discharge. Clearly, a steady frequency of discharge, $1/I$, such as that illustrated in the record of Fig. 25*a* would provide an autocorrelogram displaying a regular series of peaks in the time bins corresponding to I, $2I$, $3I$, etc., with zero count in all other bins; such an autocorrelogram is illustrated by the shaded bars of Fig. 25*c*. Record (b) of Fig. 25 was made by adding some 'randomly timed' signals to the regular signals of record (a) above. The result is, of course, an illustration of cyclical behaviour, buried in a certain amount of noise so that the cyclical aspect of the record becomes hard to detect by eye. Nevertheless, the autocorrelogram of this record (Fig. 25*c*, continuous line), shows peaks

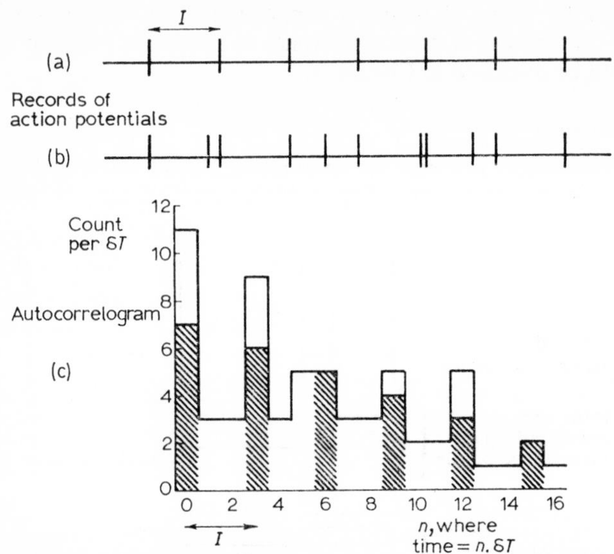

FIG. 25. The detection of cyclic behaviour by autocorrelation.
(*a*) A regular series of action potentials.
(*b*) Record constructed by adding a number of randomly timed signals to the series above.
(*c*) The autocorrelograms of records (*a*) and (*b*) above; that for (*a*) is represented by the shaded areas; that for (*b*) by the continuous line.

in the same bins as did that of Fig. 25*a*. If the record analysed had been similar, but of much greater length than the abscissa of the autocorrelogram, the latter would have shown a series of peaks of almost equal height in bins number 3, 6, 9, 12, etc. The first bin of Fig. 25*c*, for which $n \,.\, \delta T = 0$, contains a count equal to the total number of signals in the record, since every action potential can be regarded as following itself after zero time interval.

Because the autocorrelogram shows up cyclical activity, it can indicate neural feed-back of a neurone to itself; or, it can provide evidence of some cyclical drive such as regularly repeated sensory excitation. It can also be employed to discover whether a unit is responding in the same way to every one of a series of sensory stimuli or, for instance, is alternating so that it responds in a particular manner to every other stimulus.

Autocorrelograms, like interval analyses, contain information all of which is available to the experimental animal. Like the interval analysis, the autocorrelogram can also be used for determination of the functional refractory period (p. 51). In fact, the first hump of an autocorrelogram (following the empty bins that indicate functional refractory period) is usually almost identical with the first hump of an interval analysis from the same record. This is because the numbers of shortest intervals determined by both types of analysis are similar. Gerstein & Kiang (1960) have pointed out that the autocorrelogram is the sum of a number of special forms of interval analysis from the same record. Thus, if the spikes in a record are numbered consecutively 1, 2 .3, . . .

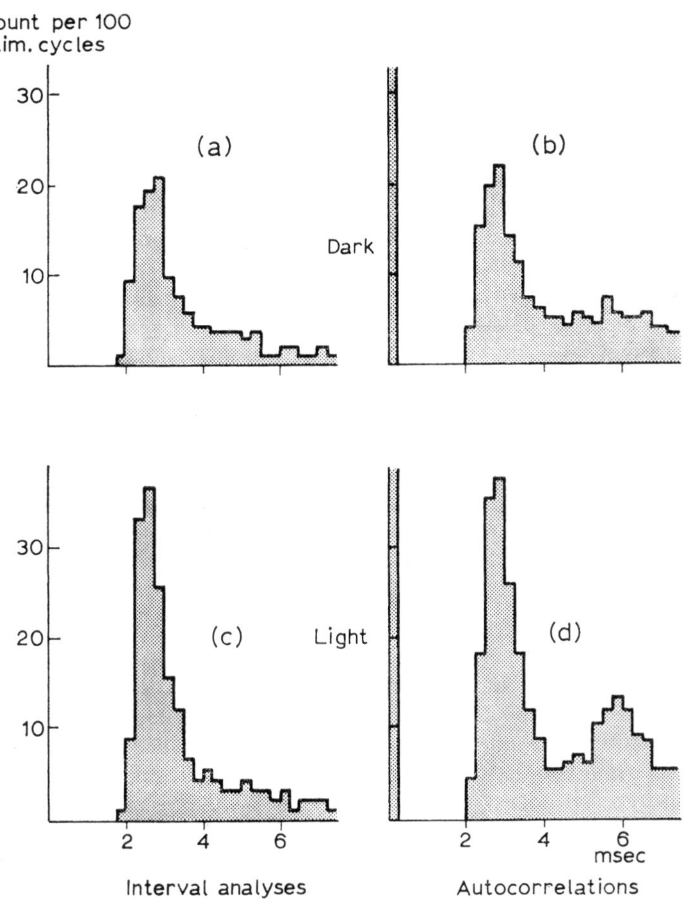

FIG. 26. Interval analyses (*a* and *c*) and autocorrelograms (*b* and *d*) from the same records of a visual unit excited by an oscillating, straight black–white border. In all cases the representative district for the neurone lay 2° from the border. For (*a*) and (*b*) it lay in the dark; for (*c*) and (*d*) the representative district was on the light side of the border.

k . . . etc., then the autocorrelation function, AC, of this record is described by:

$$AC = ID_k^{k+1} + ID_k^{k+2} + \text{etc.}$$

where ID_k^{k+1} represents the interval distribution for consecutive signals

ID_k^{k+2} represents the distribution of intervals between signals number 1 and 3, 2 and 4, 3 and 5 and so on.

While the consecutive interval analysis is easy to compute and requires relatively inexpensive equipment for automatic calculation, it contains less useful information than does the autocorrelogram. Like the interval analysis, the autocorrelogram shows the functional refractory period and indicates the mean rate of recovery of excitability; in addition, however, it can provide evidence of cyclical behaviour. Figure 26 illustrates this point, and shows two interval analyses computed for the same cell under two different physiological conditions. For the interval distribution of Fig. 26*a*, the unit was representing the dark side of a light–dark boundary in the visual field (for further details of this sort of experiment see p. 98). Figure 26*c* shows the interval analysis when the same unit was representing the light side of this border. A comparison of these two interval analyses indicates that cells representing the lighter parts of visual patterns fire with a greater number of short intervals between discharges than do the same cells representing relative darkness. Comparison of the autocorrelograms for the same two conditions (Figs. 26*b* and *d*) shows an additional fact—that only when this cell was representing the light side of a border was it likely to fire in short repetitive bursts.

Independence of the various forms of analysis

The three temporal distributions discussed above (the cross- and autocorrelograms and the consecutive interval analysis), provide three mutually independent descriptions of the same series of events. These distributions are independent in the sense that knowledge of the precise form of any two does not make prediction of the remaining one possible. Their independence is well illustrated by the results of Burns & Pritchard (1964), which are discussed at greater length in a subsequent chapter. While investigating the ways in which the position of a pattern in the visual field could alter the behaviour of neurones in the visual cerebral cortex, it was found that any one of these three temporal distributions could be altered without significant alteration in the forms of the other two.

On-line computers

It is impossible at the moment to say which aspects of the series of action potentials transmitted by a central neurone are of greatest physiological importance. One would like to know which particular parameters of unit behaviour carry information that is of critical importance in determining the responses of neighbouring neurones. Nevertheless, the distributions listed above are certainly sensitive to changes of input to the central nervous system and must presumably be closely related to physiologically important information. Moreover, these descriptions of average temporal behaviour provide information that is usually inaccessible 'by ear' or 'by eye'; a post-stimulus histogram that provides clear evidence of response to sensory stimulation can often be constructed from a record of activity, which provides no suggestion that stimuli are modifying unit behaviour, when examined with a loudspeaker or oscilloscope.

For this reason, some types of experiment become almost impossible without simultaneous (or on-line) computation. Unless one knows immediately how a neurone responded to test *A*, it is impossible to select the next test, *B*, in such a way that useful information is gained from the whole experiment. In this form of experiment, where each manoeuvre depends upon the results of preceding tests, on-line averaging is essential; without it, subsequent detailed analysis may merely show that the original experiment was poorly planned.

All the forms of temporal distribution discussed above, and many others, are readily calculated by general purpose computers, but these large and expensive instruments are not usually available for on-line work. It is for this reason that the special-purpose, small averaging computer is rapidly becoming as important in the neurophysiological laboratory as the cathode-ray oscilloscope. Unfortunately, however, the cost of such instruments is high by comparison with that of traditional neurophysiological equipment, and in assessing the merit of any on-line computer one has to take into account the number of useful analyses that it will perform per unit of price (Burns, Ferch & Mandl, 1965). Fortunately, great accuracy is not usually required in an on-line computer; records made on magnetic tape can always be analysed in detail at some later time. Consequently, considerable economy can be effected by constructing or purchasing an on-line computer that provides just sufficient accuracy to guide experimental procedure; some more exalted instrument may then be used for the final detailed measurement of records.

CHAPTER 4

THE INSTABILITY OF RANDOM NERVE NETS

THEORETICAL

Definitions

The phrase 'nerve net' implies a population of inter-connected neurones. As employed by physiologists, the term does not necessarily describe a system of cells and their interconnections that lie in one plane as do the knots of a tennis net; it is often loosely used to describe a neuronal matrix in which a system of interconnected cells occupies a volume. Defined in this way, the whole central nervous system could be regarded as one nerve net, in the sense that neuronal pathways could doubtless be traced by an enthusiastic histologist from any point within it to any other chosen point. Indeed, it would not be surprising if statistical methods ultimately demonstrated some small, but measurable, influence of any active group of neurones upon all other parts of the nervous system, however remote. On the other hand, one knows that large communities of central neurones behave in a relatively autonomous fashion. Thus, a more practical definition must involve some form of functional boundary; a nerve net could usefully be described as *a population of similar neurones which are functionally interconnected so that, when fully excitable, activity among some of them always spreads to invade the remainder*.

Fig. 27*a* illustrates a regular nerve net without feed-back. The numbered circles represent cell bodies with their associated dendrites; the arrows indicate excitatory axonal connections with neighbouring units. Clearly, if excitation spreads at all throughout the net of Fig. 27*a*, it will spread from left to right. Provided that every unit of this net is sufficiently excitable to respond to a single afferent signal, then excitation of any single neurone will cause a wave of activity to invade virtually all parts of the net to the right of the point of stimulation. If the threshold of these units is higher, so that two simultaneous incoming signals are necessary to fire any neurone, then the system will only transmit waves of excitation over a limited distance. If, for instance, cells number 1, 2 and 3 were simultaneously excited, the resulting excitation would travel no farther than unit number 9.

Networks of this sort exist in the body. Both the gut and the ureter display properties that suggest there is a neural organization of this form within their walls.

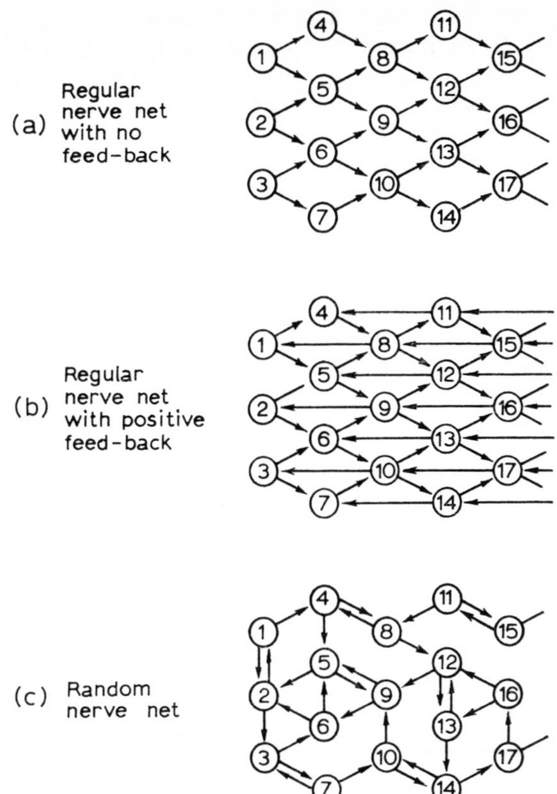

FIG. 27. Neural networks.

Figure 27*b* illustrates a regular nerve net with positive feed-back. It will be seen that this net was constructed by adding some connections to the net of Fig. 27*a* above, thus producing a network, the components of which have connections to neighbours on both left and right sides. These additional connections provide two new important properties. The network will now conduct excitation in both directions, from left to right and from right to left. The new connections also provide circuits for self-reexcitation; for instance, excitation beginning with cell number 2 will pass by way of units 5 and 6 to neurone 9; from number 9, excitation will pass back to its origin, cell 2. Thus, the system now contains positive feed-back loops which will permit reverberation, or repetitive activity on the part of their constituent neurones, so long as the circuit time exceeds the refractory period of any element making up the loop.

The system illustrated in Fig. 27*b* has many of the properties of cardiac muscle. Excitation, once started, will spread from any district to invade the whole population of cells; provided that the circuit time of the loops available for positive feed-back exceeds the refractory period of their components, excitation will always spread from its origin in an orderly fashion. Consider excitation beginning with element number 2; this will spread to invade units 5 and 6, will travel from there to units 8, 9 and 10, and so on. If the circuit time for a three-element loop such as 5, 8, 12, 5 is too short to permit self-re-excitation, then excitation will die out behind the spreading wave-front, for no larger loops than this are available. If, however, the refractory period of the elements in this syncytium were to become shorter, as is the case with cardiac muscle fibres treated with adrenaline (Goodman & Gilman, 1965), then self-reexcitation might become possible, and fibrillation would occur. Even when units in the system suffer no change of refractory period, damage of one element may precipitate the analogue of cardiac fibrillation (Lewis, 1925). If, for instance, the connections between units 5 and 9, 6 and 9 become inoperative (Fig. 27*b*), the large loop 2, 5, 8, 12, 16, 9, 2 becomes available for positive feed-back.

A random nerve net is illustrated in Fig. 27*c*. In this example, each unit can excite two neighbouring cells chosen at random. It is clear that the provision of randomly oriented excitatory interconnections, of the sort illustrated in Fig. 27*c*, necessarily gives a nerve matrix or nerve net the following properties:

1. a wave-front of excitation can travel in any direction through the system;
2. it will spread with the same velocity in all directions;
3. positive feed-back loops are available within the system for self-re-excitation.

Evidence that networks of this form are a common constituent of the mammalian central nervous system will be discussed later. Meanwhile, some reference should be made to publications which have tried to describe the properties of theoretical networks with greater precision than I have attempted in the preceding paragraphs.

Model neural networks

Beurle (1956) has considered the mathematical properties of a theoretical random network. His initial assumptions incorporated in some form many known properties of central neurones; his treatment, although less mathematically general than that of previous authors (McCulloch & Pitts, 1943; Ashby, 1950; Cragg & Temperley, 1954), is important because many of his predictions can be tested by experiment. Beurle considered a population of cells which were randomly distributed throughout a certain volume. Each unit was assumed to be connected to many of its near neighbours, and fewer of its more distant fellows, in such a way that the number of units with which it communicated declined exponentially with distance from the soma. The constants for this exponential decay in connectivity were derived from Sholl's (1953) anatomical observations of the cat's visual cerebral cortex. Beurle made the simplest possible assumptions concerning transsynaptic excitation of units within the net. He supposed that the excitatory post-synaptic potential (e.p.s.p.) was always rectangular in form and remained effective for a fixed period; he also postulated a fixed synaptic delay, defined as the time between the moment at which the summed e.p.s.p.s became effective and the time at which the excited unit initiated e.p.s.p.s upon any neighbouring cells to which it was connected. It was assumed that each cell of the network recovered full excitability suddenly and completely at a fixed time after it had been excited.

Beurle's treatment was essentially statistical in that he considered the behaviour of groups of cells rather than the responses of individual units within the system. He pointed out that properties of the net would depend critically upon the proportion of excitable cells and the fraction of 'used cells', or those that were refractory because of recent activity. It was shown that the response of the system as a whole to excitation of a small localized group of cells was all-or-nothing in nature. Weak stimuli that excite a small number of elements should produce a spreading wave of excitation that would attenuate as it travelled, and ultimately extinguish. Stronger stimuli that might excite more than a critical number of units should initiate a spreading wave of excitation that "... will increase in amplitude until it 'saturates', when it uses all the cells in the medium through which it passes, and the amplitude cannot increase further". He also showed that a wave-front of spreading excitation could leave a process of self-reexcitation in its wake. "Fully saturated waves may follow each other at intervals equal to the period taken by the cells to recover sensitivity completely, and unsaturated waves may follow even closer. This makes it possible for a wave to pass through a region, and return again to the same region some time later when the majority of the cells has recovered. This would allow a relatively local circulation of activity which might be of some importance." It is shown in the paragraphs below that there are indeed groups of cells within the central nervous system that behave in just the manner described by Beurle.

Farley & Clark (1960) have described an analogue random network, comprising 1,296 model neurones. The 'present state' of units in their network was calculated by computer and then displayed with an oscilloscope screen upon which each active neurone was indicated as a point of light within a rectangle of points representing 36×36 elements. The properties given to their model neurones were very similar to those chosen by Beurle. Farley and Clark's elements differed in possessing an excitability which recovered exponentially after the short refractory period following excitation; model excitatory post-synaptic potentials were provided with an exponential decay. Such factors as the thresholds of individual units, and the way in which connectivity varied with distance from the 'soma', were all under control of the operator. Their results include extremely elegant pictorial displays of some of Beurle's predictions. Using this method, one can witness the spread of unsaturated or saturated waves across the net. Under certain conditions, the perpetual circulation of local activity or self-reexcitation is visible. Moreover, the spread of excitation throughout the net can be halted at any moment for the instantaneous state of the units to be examined or recorded.

Farley & Clark (1960) say "For the time being . . . our approach is to use the TX-2 to generate activities by simulation, and to try varying parameters, while viewing the results, in the hope of gradually becoming 'acquainted' with the network behaviours." One hopes that this phase of empirical games with a new academic toy will soon pass, for a great deal has become known about the properties of similar neural networks in live animals since Forbes first postulated their existence in 1929. Consequently, there can be little doubt about the usefulness of such a flexible analogue net. It makes possible various quantitative predictions, concerning the behaviour of nerve nets in the live animal, that would otherwise require much tedious calculation.

RANDOM NETS IN THE NERVOUS SYSTEM

Cerebral cortex

Perhaps the most convincing evidence for the existence of central nerve nets comes from the mammalian cerebral cortex. Here, in the live animal, one can observe many of the properties that Beurle predicted for what we have called random networks. It is possible to undercut a volume of cerebral cortex in such a way that many cortical cells become neurologically isolated from the rest of the nervous system, without interference with their blood supply. In these conditions the isolated neurones retain their excitability and, provided there is no general anaesthetic present, synaptic conduction between one cell and its neighbours occurs readily. Detailed descriptions of the preparation of isolated cerebral cortex and its general properties have been given elsewhere (Burns, 1958); it is useful here, however, to summarize some of the more important findings.

Some of the cells within a slab of isolated cortex can be excited by a single artificial electrical stimulus applied to the pial surface within the isolated area. A relatively weak stimulus produces only a local response; one that spreads but attenuates as it travels and finally dies out. A stronger surface stimulus produces a wave of excitation that spreads at some 20 cm/sec to invade all parts of the isolated area. Behind the spreading wavefront, activity persists for 1–5 sec and can be recorded with a surface electrode as a series of irregular potential fluctuations, or the irregular maintained discharge of individual units can be recorded with an extracellular micro-electrode (Fig. 28). The prolonged activity

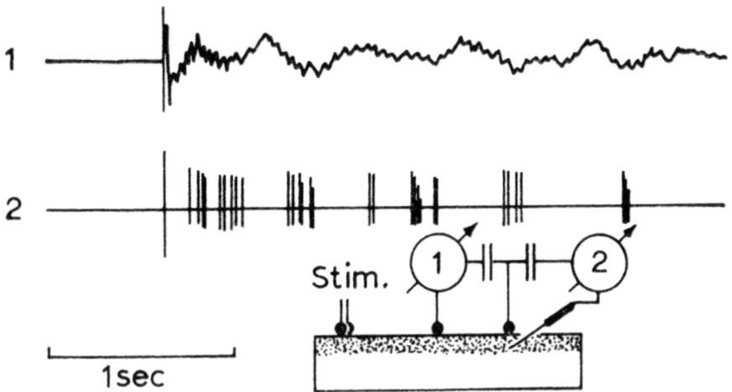

FIG. 28. Records from isolated cortex of the burst response of type B cells to a single stimulus. Records (1) and (2) were obtained simultaneously.
(Burns, 1958, *The Mammalian Cerebral Cortex*, Fig. 12, London: Edward Arnold.)

which follows individual single stimuli has been termed a burst response, for it represents a functional entity and bears an all-or-nothing relation to the strength of stimulus used for its production. A burst response can travel in any direction throughout a slab of isolated cortex and all the evidence suggests that it spreads by way of synapses. For instance, spread of this response is prevented by relatively small concentrations of general anaesthetic. Burns & Grafstein (1952) concluded that the burst response spread throughout a random network of cells and interconnecting synapses, the network being distributed as a tangential sheet about 1 mm beneath the cortical surface.

We have already pointed out that any random network should, under certain circumstances, be capable of sustained activity. It is therefore not surprising to find that each response to a single surface stimulus involves the repetitive discharge of cells within the net. If the prolonged nature of the burst response is due to the circulation of activity around loops within the net of neurones, it should be possible to prevent repetitive discharge by the application of a strong stimulus, of sufficient strength to excite simultaneously all the neurones of the network. If all units are excited simultaneously, all will become refractory at the same time and the process of self-reexcitation must stop. This prediction was tested and found to correspond with experimental results (Burns, 1951). In order that the current from a pair of surface-stimulating electrodes should have a reasonable chance of exciting all the neurones within the isolated area, a relatively small slab of isolated cortex was used. When the stimulating electrodes were near to the centre of the slab, it was found that a weak stimulus would, as usual, produce no spreading burst response; a somewhat stronger stimulus would elicit spreading and prolonged activity; stronger stimulation still produced a brief spreading response, but with no repetitive after-discharge. As would be expected, the critical stimulus strength, above which no repetitive activity was produced, was lower the nearer to the centre of the isolated area lay the stimulating electrodes (Fig. 29).

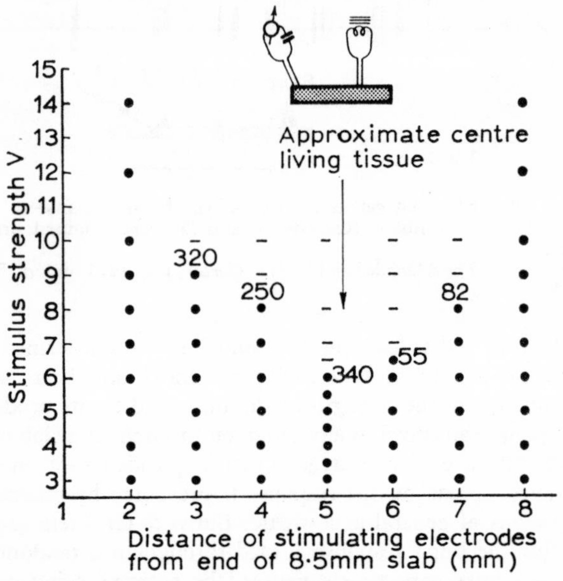

FIG. 29. Responses of a small slab of cerebral cortex (surface = $8{\cdot}5 \times 5$ mm) to single eletrical stimuli, provided at varying distances from one end of the slab. ●, prolonged surface-positive response with repetitive discharge; –, short surface-positive response with no repeating discharge. The numerical entries give the approximate latency in msec of the repetitive discharge recorded from one end of the slab.

(From Burns, 1951, *J. Physiol.*, **112,** 169, Fig. 12.)

It appears, therefore, that the process of isolating cerebral cortex reveals a system of cells, the behaviour of which conforms in every way to the properties expected of a random network.

Although the results quoted above are consistent with Beurle's predictions for excitatory random networks, it must be admitted that other explanations are possible. For instance, the strong shocks required to halt the burst response might have excited a number of inhibitory neurones which could arrest the activity of their neighbours for long enough to prevent continued self-reexcitation. Krnjevic, Randic & Straughan (1966*a*, *b*) have described a reduction in the excitability of cortical neurones which persists for 100–300 msec after a strong shock is given to the pial surface of the brain. They ascribe the silent period which follows strong surface stimulation to the action of inhibitory neurones, excited by this somewhat dramatic form of stimulation (10–100 V $\times$ 0·1 msec). In support of this contention they claim that "... these stimuli do not first excite the cells which are inhibited" and that inhibitory post-synaptic potentials (i.p.s.p.s.) can be recorded with an intracellular micropipette from most cells.

Krnjevic and his collaborators may well ultimately prove this interpretation to be correct, but the evidence provided at present is not very convincing. The prolonged membrane polarization which they interpret as a fusion of many i.p.s.p.s might well be the direct consequence of interstitial current flow caused by a stimulus of 100 V. Moreover, their own published records suggest that the inhibited cells are often first excited.

Subsequent work may force one to modify the explanation I have given of the way in which a relatively strong shock may halt the burst discharge of isolated cortical neurones. For the moment, however, it offers a simple explanation which postulates no occult phenomena and is consistent in a semi-quantitative way with Beurle's predictions.

Spinal reflex after-discharge

In many preparations set up for the recording of spinal reflex responses, a brief period of sensory excitation will induce a prolonged discharge of flexor motoneurones that far outlasts the afferent input. It was in explanation of this phenomenon that Forbes (1929) first suggested the existence of networks of interneurones, so arranged that positive feed-back was present and could maintain a process of self-reexcitation or reverberatory activity.

It is not nearly so easy to prove the presence of positive feed-back in the spinal cord as it is in the cerebral cortex where neurones are distributed in a convenient tangential sheet. Nevertheless, some properties of such a system may be tested, notably the behaviour of the preparation when provided with stimuli likely to excite a large number of the postulated interneurones simultaneously. This has been done for the reflex after-discharge of flexor motoneurones in the frog (Burns, 1956) and the results are at least consistent with Forbes' postulate. A single stimulus, applied directly to the relevant segments of the exposed spinal cord, halts the after-discharge provided that it is above a critical strength. Direct stimuli, just below this critical strength, prolong the after-discharge, which is just what would be expected if a system of neurones with positive feed-back were present. It is not possible to ascribe these effects to inhibition released by the direct stimulus, for instance by the excitation of Renshaw interneurones (Eccles, Fatt & Koketsu, 1954; Eccles, 1957), for a shock which is adequate to halt an after-discharge does not interrupt the usual sequence of events when given during sensory excitation.

These experiments suggest that Forbes was right and that spinal reflex after-discharge may be caused by positive feed-back among interneurones in the cord. Such tests require the use of experimental animals with relatively small spinal cords in order to make direct, simultaneous excitation of many interneurones possible. They should be repeated some time with such small animals as the mouse, rat or kitten.

Hunt & Kuno (1959) have examined the properties of interneurones during spinal reflex responses in the cat. They recorded the activity of individual interneurones with micro-electrodes, through which they were also able to produce direct excitation of the recorded units. They say "Self-reexcitation as the sole basis for repetitive discharge in interneurones may be ruled out by the fact that direct stimulation by a brief depolarizing pulse elicits only one impulse and no subsequent depolarization is observed. Furthermore, by weak orthodromic stimulation only a single impulse can be evoked." Their observations do not appear to me to conflict with Forbes' hypothesis. These results may simply indicate that the 'safety factor' of this nerve net is high, as it is known to be with other biological networks. The connectivity could well be so low that excitation of no single neurone within the system would be able to cause a spreading response and after-discharge. One can drive individual units in isolated cerebral cortex or in the brain stem respiratory system (see below) as fast as 500/sec by either polarizing current or injury, yet this never produces a response that spreads throughout the system.

The brain stem respiratory system

The presence of neural networks providing positive feed-back has also been postulated in that part of the brain stem which is responsible for initiating and maintaining the acts of inspiration and expiration (Burns, 1963). The bodies of nerve cells that drive respiratory motoneurones, and therefore determine the phase of respiration, lie on either side of the obex and are dispersed among other cells of the reticular formation there (Woldring & Dirken, 1951; Haber, Kohn,

Ngai, Holaday & Wang, 1957; Nelson, 1959; Salmoiraghi & Burns, 1960). Exploration of this region with a micro-electrode detects 'inspiratory cells' that provide a prolonged burst of discharges, synchronous with inspiration; in the same district, 'expiratory neurones will be found. The somata of these respiratory units are not segregated into two anatomically close-packed populations or nuclei, corresponding with the functions of inspiration and expiration. Despite the fact that cells of this system belong to one of two clearly separate functional classes, they are dispersed, apparently at random, throughout the same region (Salmoiraghi & Burns, 1960). Nevertheless, the cells of both these two functional groups appear to be connected to neighbours of

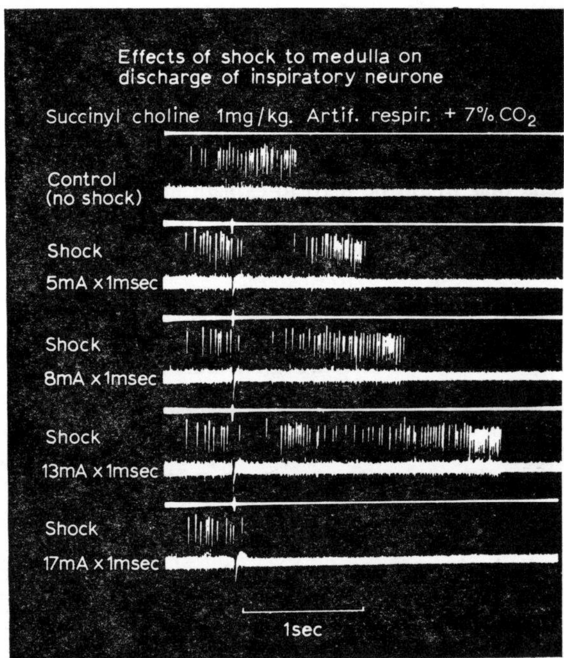

FIG. 30. Effects of shocks of progressively increasing strength given to medulla upon activity of inspiratory neurone. Anaesthetized, decerebellate, midcollicularly decerebrate, vagotomized cat paralysed with intravenous succinylcholine (1 mg/kg). Artificial ventilation with 7% CO_2 in oxygen. In each pair of records: upper trace monitors timing of shock; lower trace monitors inspiratory neurone. First pair of records from top: control (no shock). Second pair: shock of strength 5 mA; third pair: shock of strength 8 mA; fourth pair: shock of strength 13 mA; fifth pair; shock of strength 17 mA. All shocks of 1 msec duration. In all instances, stimulus triggered by first action potential of inspiratory burst after identical delays.

(From Burns & Salmoiraghi, 1960, *J. Neurophysiol.*, **23**, 27, Fig. 6.)

like function, so as to provide two neural networks, both of which exhibit evidence of positive feed-back. The two nets are interconnected by inhibitory links, so that when the neurones of one net are maximally active, members of the other net are inhibited. The evidence for positive feed-back within these two neural networks comes from experiments that are very similar to those described above with the frog's spinal cord. A strong stimulus, given to the medulla through a large electrode centred over the obex, will halt the burst of activity of either inspiratory or expiratory neurones beneath. The current strength required to bring this about is critical; stimuli of just less than critical strength prolong the burst of activity of respiratory neurones (Fig. 30). As in the case of the frog's spinal cord, these results have been interpreted as indicating that stimuli above the critical strength prevent further circulation of activity by rendering all, or a large fraction, of the relevant neurones simultaneously refractory.

Once again, the evidence for the presence of a random nerve net is not quite so convincing as it is in the case of isolated cerebral cortex. Nevertheless, the hypothesis provides a ready explanation of many phenomena that would be hard to explain in any other way. For the time being, it seems reasonable to assume that random nerve nets exist as essential functional elements in spinal cord, brain stem and cerebral cortex.

The instability of neural nets

Transmission of excitation through neural networks in the live animal is essentially stochastic in nature. When burst responses are elicited in isolated cortex by cyclically repeated, identical stimuli, no two bursts of an individual unit are exactly alike. Nor are consecutive bursts of a respiratory unit in the brain stem identical. One might argue that this lack of predictability in the temporal distribution of action potentials was due to variation of conditions outside these neural nets. For instance, the brain stem respiratory system is known to be influenced by inputs from many external sources (Burns & Salmoiraghi, 1960) which are likely to provide just that fluctuating background of tonic excitation that would account for the observed instability of respiratory neurones. In the case of isolated cortex, in which none of the neurones that can be detected with a micro-electrode appears to be active unless artificially excited, it is harder to ascribe the instability of behaviour to influences that are external to the type B network. One would have to search for evidence of slight movement of the stimulating electrodes, imperfect neural isolation, or perhaps variations of local blood supply.

It seems much more likely that the stochastic behaviour of cells within these nets is produced by uncertainty of synaptic transmission across the many interneural junctions that are involved. It is usually assumed that transmission of excitation between one central neurone and its neighbour is humoral and consequently similar in many respects to transmission from motoneurone to skeletal muscle. If this is so, one might expect a certain random leakage of transmitter, such as that first detected by Fatt & Katz (1952) at the neuromuscular junction (p. 21). At this peripheral site, leakage of transmitter does not lead to uncertainty of transmission because each action potential of the motoneurone liberates far more transmitter than is normally necessary to excite a muscle fibre; most central neurones, however, are designed to respond, by spatial summation, only to simultaneous excitation arriving by many afferent pathways. Consequently, one might expect to find that response of any central unit to a specific set of inputs was stochastic in nature. These considerations make the observed uncertainties of transmission across neural nets somewhat less surprising.

There is, in fact, some evidence in support of the argument given above. In isolated cortex it is possible to excite type **B** units through a subcortical pathway by using white matter below the relevant neurone. In these circumstances, a stimulus strength that is submaximal for the burst response can be found that will sometimes elicit a response from the nerve cell, and sometimes will not. But it can, of course, still be argued that this unpredictability of response is due to inconstancy of afferent excitation, due either to minute movements of the subcortical-stimulating electrodes or perhaps to small variations in excitability of nerve fibres accessible to the stimulating current.

Function of random nets in the nervous system

The finding that random nerve nets may exist in districts of the nervous system as far apart as cerebral cortex, brain stem and spinal cord, immediately suggests that this particular organization of neurones must provide functional characteristics of considerable importance. In order to explain the popularity of this component of the nervous system, one should perhaps seek properties whose value outweighs the fact that a nerve net is a relatively expensive unit in terms of number and volume of neurones.

The all-or-nothing relationship between magnitude of input and the spread of activity provides a barrier to the weak stimulus. The observation that maximal excitation of one unit within these nets (at least in the cerebral cortex and respiratory system) does not excite the rest of the population, provides evidence for a reasonable safety factor. It implies that the networks are protected from excitation by a fortuitously high frequency of discharge in any one afferent fibre. For afferent excitation to have access through the network to other parts of the nervous system, the input must exceed a certain threshold which is dependent upon a sufficiently frequent discharge, in an adequate number of afferent fibres, reaching the net with a sufficient local, anatomical density. Provided this threshold is exceeded, excitation will spread throughout all excitable parts of the net, monopolizing it so that the functional access of rival inputs is temporarily blocked.

One can readily visualize the usefulness of such an arrangement to cerebral cortex and spinal cord. There will be no transmission of stimuli that are weak in terms of local density and frequency of afferent signals; on the other hand, suprathreshold excitation will be given infinite amplification and transmitted, whatever the nature of subsequent inputs. It is presumably this infinite amplification that 'justifies the use of random neural nets' in a system providing respiratory drive. Positive feed-back is a necessary element in the construction of any bistable system; moreover, the respiratory drive requires, in addition to alternate inspiration and expiration, that each phase of activity should be sufficient in magnitude and duration for tidal air to exceed the dead space. Thus, the reciprocally connected neural nets that form the brain stem respiratory system ensure that, when necessary, respiration is diminished by reduction in the frequency of movements without dangerous reduction of their amplitude.

The presence of a widespread, tangentially oriented, neural net in the cerebral cortex, provides a system capable of conducting excitation over great distances. It offers a physiological explanation of the observation from experimental psychology, that appropriate training can form connections between virtually any sensory input and any motor output. Transmission of burst responses can be demonstrated in slabs of cortex isolated from auditory, visual and parietal cortex. The type B network (Burns & Grafstein, 1952) is either spread all over the cortex or at least covers the larger part of the brain's surface. It is not, of course, suggested that transmission occurs solely within the cortical grey matter. The known velocity of transmission for the burst response (about 20 cm/sec) is far too slow to account for reaction times of the order of 150 msec. It is possible, of course, that transmission throughout the same network, operating in intact cortex, is considerably faster since a constant input from subcortical fibres may increase the excitability of its constituent neurones. It seems more likely, however, that cortico-cortical fibres play an important role in speeding conduction by short-circuiting a system of cortical synapses that is essential to transmission. This postulate is consistent with Sperry, Miner & Myers (1955) finding that multiple subpial incisions of the visual cortex did not interfere measurably with acquired behaviour, provided that these cuts did not involve the subcortical white matter.

The sheet of interconnected cells that gives rise to the burst response of isolated cortex is clearly capable of conducting excitation for very great distances across the surface of the brain. Admittedly, nothing resembling the burst response of isolated cortex is seen in the intact unanaesthetized forebrain, but presumably in this case the activity of type B cells is modified by extracortical influences. Beurle showed (1956) in his theoretical discussion of such networks that the spatio-temporal pattern of waves spreading from an excited focus would be modified by the presence of other inputs to the net. One has to assume that the network is operating in intact brain and that the same cell junctions as conduct the burst response of isolated cortex are available to the spread of normal patterns of activity (Burns, 1958). For the moment, it seems reasonable to assume that the type B cell network plays a significant role in the conduction of excitation from one part of the brain to another. If this is so, it becomes important to know what types of information can be transmitted by this net, and in what ways this information may be modified in transit.

One might expect such a network to transmit information concerning the site and temporal nature of local excitation. In fact, the burst response of isolated cortex appears to convey rather little information about either. It is true that the average temporal pattern of firing during the burst discharge of any unit within the net is to some extent dependent upon the site of excitation within a slab of isolated cortex (Burns, 1958). The post-stimulus histograms obtained from the bursts of a type B cell in response to exciting a slab of isolated cortex with surface electrodes at two different places are shown in Figs. 31*a* and *b*. Figure 31*a* shows the average response to 100 stimuli given to site *A* at 1/1·6 sec.; Fig. 31*b* represents the response to 100 similar stimuli, given at site *B*, 12 mm from site *A*. The difference between these two histograms is not impressive and it seems that the uncertain or stochastic nature of transmission across the interneural junctions of this net does not permit the passage of much information concerning the site of excitation within the network.

The burst response appears to convey somewhat more information about the relatively low frequency characteristics of remote excitation. The histogram of Fig. 31*c* was obtained by averaging the response to 100 stimuli given to site *B* at 1/sec; it shows some difference in shape from Fig. 31*b* which was obtained by delivering the same stimuli to the same place at 1/1·6 sec. Nevertheless, the type B network carries virtually no information about the high-frequency aspects of stimulation. The shapes of the histograms in Figs. 32*a* and *b* are very similar, although they were generated by stimulating at 1/1·6 sec the same point with 100 bursts of 5 stimuli at 50/sec, and 5 stimuli at 100/sec respectively.

It seems that the widespread, tangentially oriented network of type B cells is not well adapted for the transmission of information concerning either the exact site or the high frequency characteristics

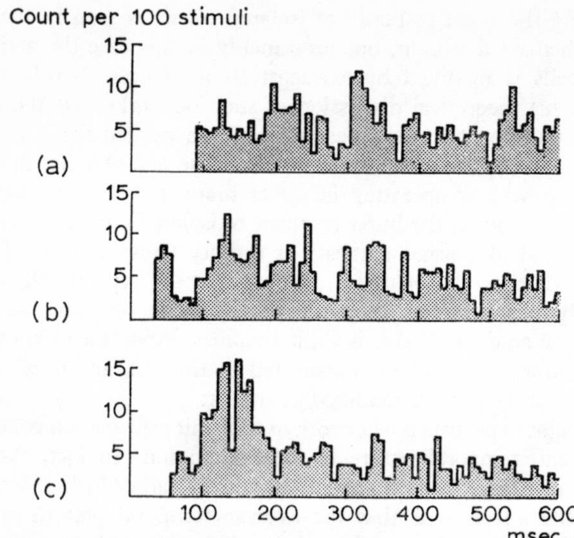

FIG. 31. Post-stimulus histograms from a type B unit in parietal, isolated cerebral cortex.

(*a*) The average response to 100 single stimuli given once in 1·6 sec to point *A* on the surface of 15 mm slab, at one end.

(*b*) The average response to 100 single stimuli given once in 1·6 sec to point *B*, 12 mm from point *A* and at the opposite end of the slab's surface.

(*c*) Response to the same stimulation of point *B*, but given at 1/sec.

of inputs to the net. Farley & Clark (1960) have pointed out that ". . . a net of these elements has the property of transforming timed stimuli . . . into spatial patterns of active elements and (if a suitable time is chosen) that the transformation may be unique". In the case of the type B net, the suitable time appears to be greater than 50/sec. This observation may imply that the top end of the mammalian nervous system is 'uninterested' in the high-frequency characteristics of afferent inputs, except in so far as these are one indication of the biological strength of an incoming signal.

On the other hand, the type B net is well adapted for:

a. the rejection of weak inputs,
b. response to inputs that are strong with respect to number of active afferent fibres and frequency of discharge of these fibres.

It can transmit the information that a suprathreshold stimulus has occurred, without apparently indicating the instantaneous strength of the input. It will indicate something of the low-frequency characteristics

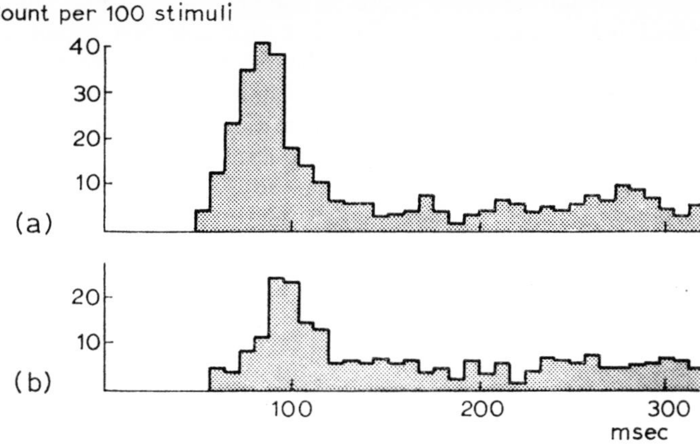

FIG. 32. Post-stimulus histograms from the same unit as that providing Fig. 31.

(*a*) The average response to 100 bursts of stimuli, each consisting of 5 stimuli at 50/sec, repeated once every 1·6 sec. The stimuli were given at point *B* on the slab's surface and were of the same strength as those providing Fig. 31 b.

(*b*) The average response to the same stimulus given in bursts of 5 at 100/sec.

In both graphs, time is measured along the abscissa from the last stimulus of the average burst.

of remote excitation, thereby converting temporal to spatial patterns. Moreover, the direction of tangential spread of the wave-front of excitation will be determined by the spatial distribution of local inputs that have recently been active, for it has been shown that type B cells remain super-excitable for many minutes after each burst discharge (Burns, 1951, 1958). Thus the network can transmit information about the site and sequence of recent suprathreshold inputs. Because of the stochastic nature of interneural transmission, and because of the high safety factor, to which we have already referred, the network will maintain its properties despite the loss or malfunction of individual units. One can readily visualize the importance of this built-in redundancy to the normal function of both cerebral cortex and brain stem respiratory system.

The whole brain regarded as a nerve net

There are some advantages in regarding the whole forebrain as one immense nerve net, composed of many units with relatively similar properties. Such an approach has the merit that it makes no unjustified assumptions about the functional implications of neuro-anatomy, which has so far proved singularly unhelpful in providing an intelligible concept of brain function. Smith & Smith (1965), whose work is described below, argued "that the most profitable first approach to cortical mechanisms may be to regard the tissue as composed of a small number of functional elements reiterated uniformly and to regard the various classical subdivisions of the cortex as regions in which connections to or from other parts of the brain occur with greatest density. While it is recognized that to ignore the obvious histological and physiological differences from one area to another may lead to dangerous oversimplification, nevertheless such an approach might well reveal general properties of cortical physiology which would otherwise have been overlooked, and lead to generalizations which can be applied to the specific conditions of connection in each part of cortex."

Burns & Smith (1962) made successful use of this non-anatomical and statistical approach in their investigations of spread of activity through the unanaesthetized cat's brain. Further reference to their work is made on p. 115. Smith & Smith (1965) have used a similar approach in their attempt to analyse the nature of spontaneous activity in the isolated, unanaesthetized forebrain. In a good preparation of this sort, where the forebrain has been separated from the rest of the nervous system by an intercollicular cut, which does not interfere with the basilar blood supply, all nerve cells that can be detected by an extracellular micropipette exhibit continual 'spontaneous' activity. Various average rates of unit discharge are encountered, between some 5 and 30/sec, but the most common rate is around 10/sec.

Despite many investigations, the cause of this continual activity is still obscure. Although there is a high level of excitability, no cells in isolated cerebral cortex show convincing evidence of 'spontaneous' activity, in the cardiac sense of the word. It seems that the periodic discharge of cortical cells in the intact cerebral cortex must be excited by activity originating outside the cortical grey matter (see Burns, 1958). There may, of course, be neurones in the upper brain stem capable of spontaneous discharge, and one must remember that the isolated forebrain has two sensory pathways intact—those from the eye and the nose. Very little activity on the part of any pacemaker that there may be would be necessary to maintain the observed continual activity of cortical neurones, for it has been shown that after-bursts may continue for many minutes following focal excitation of isolated cortex; moreover, Burns & Smith (1962) have shown that the disturbance transmitted from a single, focal, cortical stimulus in the whole brain, lasts for some 5 seconds. Whatever the correct explanation of continual activity in the isolated forebrain, it seems safe to assume that cortical cells only discharge in response to afferent excitation by their neighbours.

It is difficult to be sure how many independent afferent pathways converge upon the average cortical cell; it seems, however, that this number is likely to be about 2,000. For the visual cortex of the cat, Sholl (1956) provides the following estimates:

a. fibres, afferent to the cortex	25,000/mm^2
b. fibres, efferent from the cortex	75,000/mm^2
c. density of neurones	72,000/mm^3
d. thickness of cortex	1·75 mm

He also believes that one afferent fibre, ascending to the visual cortex from the lateral geniculate body, makes functional contact with some 5000 cortical units. If all fibres carrying excitation into the cortex connect with a similar number of units, one can estimate the number of pathways feeding each unit as in the region of:

$$\frac{25{,}000 \times 5000}{72 \times 1750} \simeq 1000$$

Only about half the neurones in the cortex give rise to axons that leave the grey matter; if the anatomical connectivity of the remaining units with their neighbours is of the same order as that of subcortical afferent fibre, we should estimate the number of afferent paths feeding the average cortical cell as in the region of 2000. Such estimates of convergence are extremely inaccurate, but suffice to show that the number of independent sources of excitation for a cortical neurone is probably very large.

With a large number of independent excitatory inputs, one would expect the times of discharge of a cortical cell to be random with respect to time, whatever the temporal pattern of the independent inputs. The distribution of intervals between action potentials should be exponential.

Smith & Smith (1965) found that this was not so; spontaneously active cortical units tended to fire in bursts more or less clearly separated by relatively long intervals of inactivity. The 40 spontaneously active cortical neurones that they examined all showed interval distributions that were not exponential, but exhibited a "preponderance of short intervals with a long right-hand 'tail' indicating the presence of a small number of very long intervals". The distributions obtained from most of these cells could be fitted by assuming that the observed interspike intervals represented the sum of two exponential distributions (Fig. 33). Their records were interpreted as showing that all cortical cells were controlled by two apparently independent processes; a 'fast' process providing random excitation at relatively high frequency, that was gated on and off by a 'slow' process. For the majority of the cells examined, the times of opening and closure of the gate were random with respect to time. When the mean frequency of a spontaneously active cell was increased by a period of tip-negative unit polarization

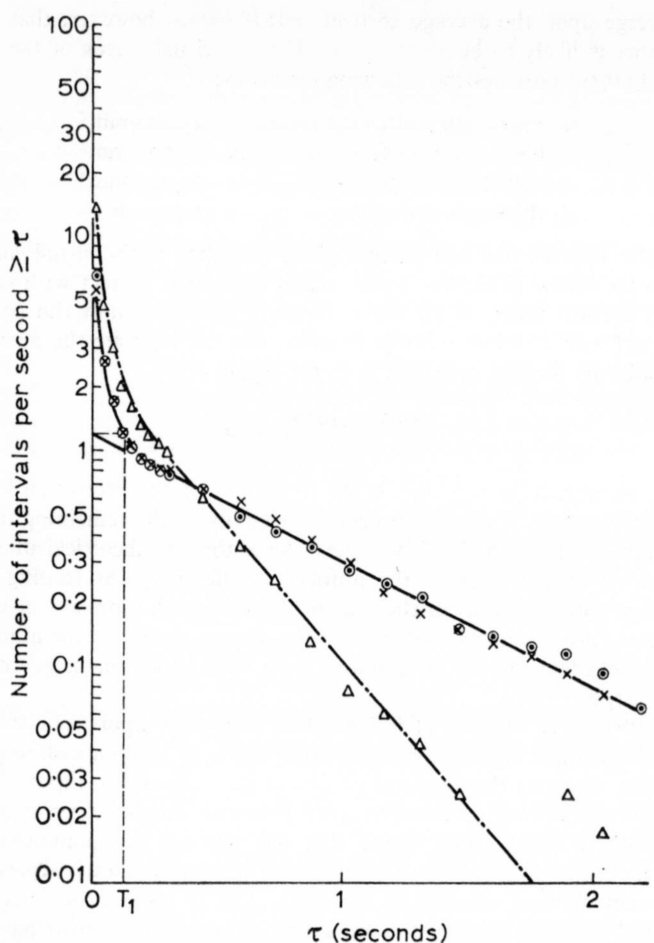

FIG. 33. Interpulse interval distributions obtained from a cell in the median suprasylvian gyrus. The crosses (x) are from a 216 sec sample of 'spontaneous' firing in the unstimulated brain. The effect of passing −0·2 μa for 120 sec through the pipette tip (Δ) was to increase the average firing rate from 5·5 pulses/sec to 13·4 pulses/sec. After the removal of polarization (⊙) the distribution reverts to the original form (109 sec sample).

(From Smith & Smith, 1965, *Biophys. J.*, **5**, 47, Fig. 2.)

(see p. 153), the Smiths' 'slow' process was reversibly changed without alteration of their 'fast' process (Fig. 33).

It seems reasonable to assume that tip-negative current flow through the recording electrode will produce local depolarization and will consequently lower a neurone's threshold to incoming excitation (see also p. 155). The observed rise in mean frequency is consistent with this interpretation. But the apparent independence of the fast and slow processes in the face of local polarizing currents would seem to imply different sites of control by these two mechanisms. One possible explanation of this finding would be to suppose that the 'gating' or slow process played only upon the somata of neurones, which is probably that part most affected by the passage of current through a micropipette that has been placed for satisfactory recording. On this view, the excitation provided by the fast process would mostly arise in dendritic structures beyond the reach of polarizing current. The recent results of Anderson & Lømo (1965) are consistent with this hypothesis. Records from electrodes inside the somata of pyramidal neurones in the hippocampus of the rabbit have shown that spikes can be generated without any recordable somatic e.p.s.p. by afferent volleys; nevertheless, the afferent volleys produced large negative field-potentials that could be recorded with extracellular electrodes in the vicinity of the activated dendritic synapses. They believed that their results indicated "... a dendritic origin of the synaptically induced action potentials of the pyramidal neurones".

The measurement of predictability

While discussing the behaviour of nerve nets in the live animal, we have encountered several systems that show different degrees of predictability. The behaviour of a single cell in the isolated, intact forebrain of the unanaesthetized cat is much less predictable than is the behaviour of an inspiratory neurone of the brain stem during spontaneous respiration of the same animal. Type B neurones, during the burst response of isolated cerebral cortex, exhibit an even greater irregularity of behaviour. While it is sometimes easy to classify orders of irregularity, as in the case of the first two of these examples, it is useful to have some objective and numerical measure of predictability, or its converse—uncertainty. For example, one might ask, "Does the behaviour of an inspiratory neurone belonging to the brain stem respiratory system become more regular as the pCO_2 of the blood is increased? What change in regularity is associated with unit alteration of pCO_2?" In this case, it would immediately become necessary to define predictability and specify a little more precisely exactly what must be predicted. If interest were focused upon the intervals between consecutive acts of inspiration, then some measure would have to be found for dispersion among the longest intervals between discharges of the respiratory unit, since a long interval precedes the first action potential of each burst of inspiratory activity. If one were more interested in predictability of behaviour during the burst of a respiratory unit, then it might be useful to compute the average temporal distribution of action potentials following the first discharge of each burst (a form of analysis that would be similar to the construction of a post-stimulus histogram).

Various measures of predictability have been described. The estimate of 'response', used by Burns & Smith (1962), is essentially a measure of predictability in relation to an artificial stimulus. This measure is referred to in more detail on pp. 46–47. When examining the behaviour of somatic sensory neurones in the thalamus, Poggio & Vierstein (1964) used the Poisson model as a reference for estimating predictability. Predictability was defined by them in terms of deviation from the interval distribution expected from a Poisson series (see Fig. 23*b*). However, in addition to many obvious disadvantages, such a definition would fail to measure the perfect predictability of the series of signals illustrated in Fig. 34 and described below.

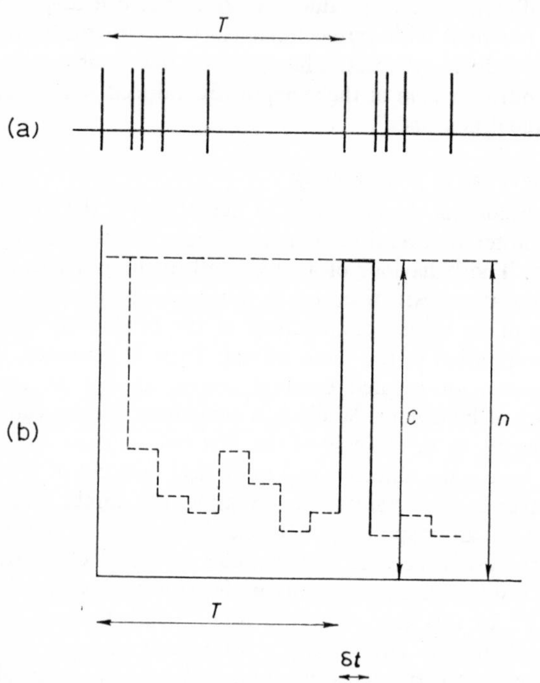

FIG. 34. Illustrating the measurement of predictability (see text).

Consider an endless series of impulses, such as the spikes recorded from a central neurone with an extracellular micro-electrode. One might ask, "If observation of this series of signals were to cease suddenly at some specified point after a long period of observation, what would be the most accurate statement that could be made about the timing of any subsequent signal?" If observation were terminated after any signal of the series, an observer might say, "The most probable time for one of the next signals will be between T and $T+\delta t$ after the last signal that I witnessed. The signal should occur here with a probability, P." The accuracy of this statement could be measured as

$$A = \frac{P(T-\delta t)}{T}$$

which is dimensionless and can vary between zero and unity (provided, of course, that $0 \leqslant \delta t \leqslant T$ and $T \neq 0$).

Figure 34*a* shows a temporal pattern of signals that is repeated cyclically with a mean frequency of $1/T$. The two identical bursts of activity shown are supposed to illustrate random firing within the burst. The autocorrelogram for such a series will show a count, C, for the interval between T and $(T+\delta t)$, which equals the total number of signals, n, used for its computation (Fig. 34*b*). Thus, if such a series were stopped at any individual signal, an observer could predict that the most probable time for the next signal would be between T and $(T+\delta t)$, where it would occur with a probability of $P=C/n$. In this case, C, the greatest count in any bin, must equal n, however small δt is chosen. Therefore an observer could make a statement about the next signal, of the greatest possible accuracy; i.e. $A=1$. This would, of course, not be true if the intervals between identical bursts of activity were not all equal to the same value, T; then the series would only be perfectly predictable in relation to the first discharge of each burst.

Accuracy of prediction, A, as defined above, must vary with the choice of δt. This fact may be made clearer by consideration of a series of signals such as that shown in Fig. 35. In this series the intervals between consecutive spikes are supposed to be nearly, but not quite, constant. If a value for δt were chosen that was larger than the variation between intervals, then C as determined from the autocorrelogram would equal n, the total count, and P would be estimated as unity. If, however, δt had been chosen smaller than the variation of intervals between signals, then C_1 (Fig. 35*b*), the largest count in any bin, would have been less than n, and P would have been estimated as less than unity. Thus, to provide an estimate of maximal predictability, one clearly needs to find a value for δt that brings C nearest to n, without at the same time introducing too much indeterminacy into the predicted timing of the most probable signal. Referring again to Fig. 35*b*, the greatest value of C is C_1. But had we taken δt three times larger, the maximum value of C would have been $C_1+C_2+C_3=n$.

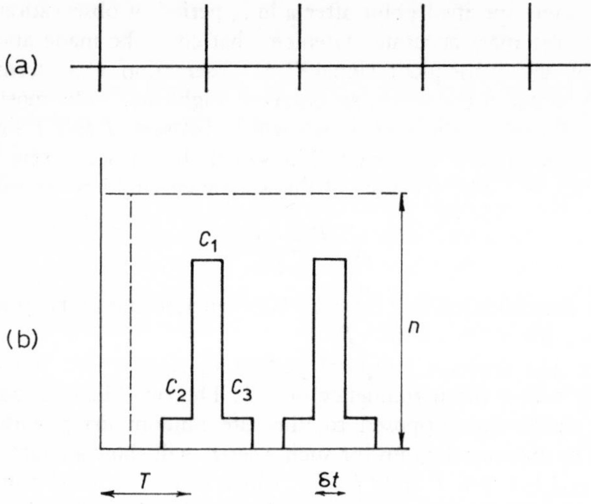

FIG. 35. Illustrating the dependence of predictability upon choice of δt (see text).

A useful definition of predictability might run as follows: *An observer is suddenly prevented from seeing a continuous series of signals, after a large number of signals,* n, *has occurred with a mean frequency,* f. *Predictability for this series is the maximum accuracy with which the observer could predict correctly any future signal, where none would have been expected from a knowledge of* f *alone.* To estimate predictability, P_R, according to this definition, one must search for the maximum value of:

$$A \times (\text{probability that a spike would not have occurred by chance in the chosen interval } \delta t)$$

A time bin, δt, must be selected for the formation of an autocorrelogram, such that it is less than the shortest interval between signals (or such that the probability of two signals within δt is extremely small). A knowledge of the mean frequency, f, tells one that the chance of a signal falling within any chosen δt, is $f \times \delta t$. The chance of a chosen δt containing no signal, calculated from a knowledge of the mean frequency, is $(1 - f \,.\, \delta t)$. Likewise, the chance that no signal will occur in any of N consecutive intervals of δt, will be $(1 - f \,.\, N \,.\, \delta t)$. Thus, maximum predictability for the series would be estimated by searching for the maximum value of:

$$\frac{(C_1 + C_2 + \ldots C_N)}{n} \times (1 - f \,.\, N \,.\, \delta t) \times \left(\frac{T - N \,.\, \delta t}{T}\right)$$

where C_1, C_2, etc., are the largest neighbouring counts in the vicinity of the greatest peak in the autocorrelogram, occurring at time, T. This estimate is dimensionless and can vary between zero and unity.

Where predictability with respect to any signal is required, n will refer to the total number of signals contributing to the autocorrelogram. If predictability with respect to a stimulus or to the first action potential of a burst is needed, then the average temporal distribution following the reference signal (stimulus or first discharge) must be computed. C_1, C_2, etc., will refer to counts in the histogram of this distribution, and n will be entered as the number of reference signals used in the computation. Table 1 provides estimates of predictability obtained in this way for some central units in unanaesthetized cats.

TABLE 1

Predictability of units in the unanaesthetized cat

Unit location	*T, sec*	*Predictability*
Brain stem inspiratory neurone (decerebrate preparation)	3·7	0·69
Same, within individual bursts	0·036	0·40
In visual cortex when 'driven' by visual pattern given artificial saccades at irregular frequency (isolated forebrain)	0·004	0·089
Same visual unit during spontaneous activity	0·004	0·065
Type B unit in isolated parietal cerebral cortex	0·0045	0·056

CHAPTER 5

THE UNCERTAIN RESPONSE OF CORTICAL NEURONES

THE continual activity of cortical neurones in the unanaesthetized brain has been referred to in the preceding chapter. Although the precise times of firing of a cortical unit are unpredictable, the mean number of discharges per minute remains remarkably constant for long periods of time provided that the nervous system is undisturbed (Burns, Heron & Pritchard, 1962; Bindman, Lippold & Redfearn, 1964). Sensory excitation can alter this mean firing rate (Mountcastle, Davies & Berman, 1957; Burns, Heron & Pritchard, 1962), but more often simply causes a redistribution of the times of discharge without any significant change of mean frequency. For instance, in the visual cortex, most units display an increased probability of discharge soon after the ON or OFF of appropriately placed retinal illumination; but the probability of discharge at other times during the cycle of retinal excitation is reduced, so that the net frequency remains the same as the 'spontaneous' value, when no sensory excitation is provided (Burns, Heron & Pritchard, 1962). We have also pointed out (Chapter 3) the stochastic nature of such responses and the fact that any quantitative relation between stimulus and response must be given in statistical terms.

These observations may imply that the average firing frequency of cortical neurones is a relatively unimportant aspect of their behaviour, but do not tell one which parameters of the average response are physiologically important, in that they determine the behaviour of other cells in the central nervous system. The paragraphs below represent an attempt to answer three questions, all of which are concerned with the code in which neurones of the sensory cortex may represent events in the animal's environment:

a. What sort of input to cortical neurones most readily excites them?
b. How is the external world represented in sensory cortex? By what sorts of code of neural behaviour?
c. What is transmitted from the neurones of sensory cortex, for use by the rest of the brain?

Most of the available information on these points comes from experiments on the mammalian visual system, because it has proved relatively easy to control. If one wishes to generalize, it is necessary at present to assume that those properties of the central visual response which are of physiological importance have their counterpart in other sensory systems. Later experience with the somatic and auditory systems may force us to qualify or abandon this assumption; but for the time being it seems sensible to assume that the nervous system will make use of only a small number of neural codes, and will exhibit in this respect the same sort of economy that is apparent for types of cells and for their simpler functions.

THE EXCITATION OF CORTICAL NEURONES

Cortical neurones, like spinal motoneurones, presumably make use of spatial and temporal summation to sort and select afferent excitation for rejection or further transmission. It was pointed out, in the preceding chapter, that excitation of one unit in a neural network never produces a spreading response. This resistance to activation by the maximal firing of one unit certainly provides a useful safety factor for the system, but is also a necessary property of units which must sort incoming stimuli by spatial summation. Because they are designed for temporal summation, cortical neurones show a similar resistance to excitation by single afferent volleys. Burns & Smith (1962) used various forms of cortical stimulation when studying the spread of excitation through the brain. They found that single stimuli, applied directly to the cortical surface, were much less efficient in producing a spreading response than were short bursts of similar stimuli. A burst of ten stimuli given to the pial surface of the brain at 100/sec proved to be a useful form of artificial stimulation. During the same series of experiments it was also found that physiological forms of cortical stimulation, such as that produced by a flash of light on the retina or a click-stimulus to the ear, were more efficient in producing a spreading response than was any form of direct cortical stimulus. Input to the cortex from the optic radiations certainly consists in bursts of action potentials rather than individual signals (Bishop, Burke & Davis, 1959; Hubel & Wiesel, 1961); moreover, unlike artificial direct stimulation, physiological excitation provides a form of input which cortical units have seen before. Burns & Bliss (unpublished) working with slabs of isolated cortex, which were excited by fine electrodes thrust into the subcortical white matter, found it far easier to fire cortical units with short bursts of high-frequency stimulation than it was with single volleys. In relation to this question of temporal summation, it is interesting to note that Pinsky & Burns (1962) found that artificial direct cortical stimulation at some 50/sec was more effective in producing epileptiform after-discharge than was any other frequency of excitation.

Cells in the visual cortex are more likely to be excited by local retinal stimuli than by diffuse retinal illumination (Hubel & Wiesel, 1959, 1962); this is partly due to the fact that ganglion cells of the retina show the same preference for local illumination. Kuffler has shown (1953) that ganglion cells in the cat have circular receptive fields, the field consisting of two parts: a central circular area within which illumination of a small area produces an ON response, and a concentric outer field where the same stimulus proves to be inhibitory; in this case, the OFF of a peripheral stimulus would be excitatory. Thus, such a ganglion cell would be described as having a circular receptive field that was ON-centre and OFF-periphery; other ganglion cells show OFF-centres with ON-peripheries. The lateral inhibition implied by this arrangement ensures that local retinal stimuli will be more exciting to optic nerve fibres than will diffuse illumination (Kuffler, Fitzhugh & Barlow, 1957). There appears to be no substantial reorganization of signals as they pass through the lateral geniculate body. Extracellular recordings from the somata of lateral geniculate neurones have shown concentric, circular receptive fields that are very similar to those of ganglion cells—ON-centre with OFF-periphery, or vice versa (Hubel & Wiesel, 1961). There was some evidence that passage through the lateral geniculate body increased the amount of lateral inhibition; the ability of a peripheral receptive field to inhibit the centre response was more marked for geniculate cells than it was for fibres of the optic nerve.

The receptive fields for cells in the visual cortex are similar, showing mutually inhibitory districts, but they are not circular (Hubel & Wiesel, 1962). Hubel and Wiesel found that "For cortical cells, specifically oriented lines and borders tend to replace circular spots as the optimal stimuli, movement becomes an important parameter of stimulation, diffuse light becomes virtually ineffective . . .". All who have worked on the visual system in the rabbit, cat and monkey are agreed that there is a point-to-point correspondence between directions in the visual field and districts of maximal excitation in the visual cortex (Hubel, 1963). Therefore, the observation that local retinal stimuli provide the most effective excitation of cortical cells implies that a localized input to the cortex from the optic radiations is more exciting than a diffuse input. A similar, but less dramatic, form of receptive field appears to obtain in the somatic sensory cortex, for Mountcastle (1957) said, "Our observations indicate the disposition of inhibitory fields for cortical cells which surround their excitatory fields. Thus a single stimulated point" (physiological excitation of peripheral sensory end-organs) "producing a cortical cell discharge zone, will inhibit the surrounding cortical areas." All these observations suggest that units in the cerebral cortex are more readily excited by local inputs than by the arrival of spatially dispersed afferent signals.

In general, it is change in the environment rather than steady environmental state that determines reaction of the nervous system. It is not surprising therefore to find that in many cortical districts units are most excited by alterations of sensory input and appear to disregard steady states. There are many modalities of sensation for which accommodation of peripheral receptors removes information about the steady state of the environment from the afferent input to the nervous system; but in the case of proprioception, hearing and sight, this is not always the case. Nevertheless, cortical neurones concerned with the registration of light and sound appear to respond best to changes of sensory input. All of the many investigations of cortical response to retinal excitation have employed either flashing or moving light as a stimulus because no response to stationary, continuous illumination could be detected. Cortical units that will respond clearly to flashing or moving retinal patterns, as judged by the post-stimulus histogram, show no sign of response to stationary, continuous illumination. After a brief ON response at the presentation of light, continuous illumination produces no measurable deviation from the spontaneous activity recorded in the dark; the mean frequency of units remains unchanged (Burns, Heron & Pritchard, 1962), and there is no measurable alteration of interval distribution or autocorrelation. This observation is consistent with the findings of experimental human psychology, already referred to (p. 30), which have indicated a loss of normal perception for the stabilized image. On the other hand, it is known that mammalian optic nerve fibres feed the central nervous system with continual information about the steady state of retinal illumination (Kuffler, Fitzhugh & Barlow, 1957); this information is probably used by the brain stem for the control of pupillary diameter, but apparently does not influence the behaviour of neurones in the cerebral cortex. At this level, units are only affected by local change in retinal illumination.

Patterns focused upon the cat's retina appear to be most exciting to the visual cortex, when provided with an oscillatory movement at about 3 c/s and an amplitude of some 50 min arc. The unanaesthetized, isolated forebrain of the cat provides a very convenient preparation for the study of central responses to patterned retinal excitation. However, since the physiological nystagmus of the intact animal is absent in this preparation (Pritchard & Heron, 1960), patterns must be either flashed or moved across the retina to excite units in the visual cortex. Consequently, it is important from both a theoretical and a technical point of view, to determine the most efficient form of stimulation that corresponds as closely as possible to normal retinal excitation in the intact animal. Burns, Heron & Pritchard (1962) projected a straight, black-white border upon the retina and provided this simple pattern with 'artificial saccadic movements' consisting in a rectangular cyclic oscillation, perpendicular to the border. Both amplitude and frequency of oscillation could be varied. All of the cortical units studied showed a maximal response at 3 c/s (Fig. 36) while the efficiency of excitation

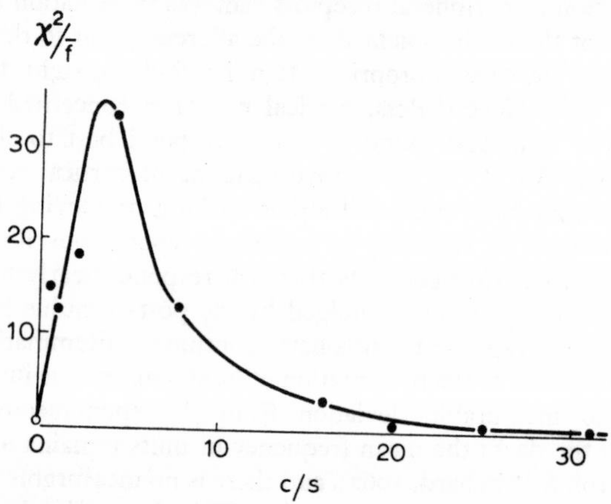

FIG. 36. Responses (ordinate) of a cortical neurone to retinal excitation by horizontal light–dark boundary oscillating at various frequencies (abscissa). Amplitude 50 min arc.
(From Burns, Heron & Pritchard, 1962, *J. Neurophysiol.*, **25**, 165, Fig. 7.)

increased with amplitude, up to some 50 min arc (Fig. 37).

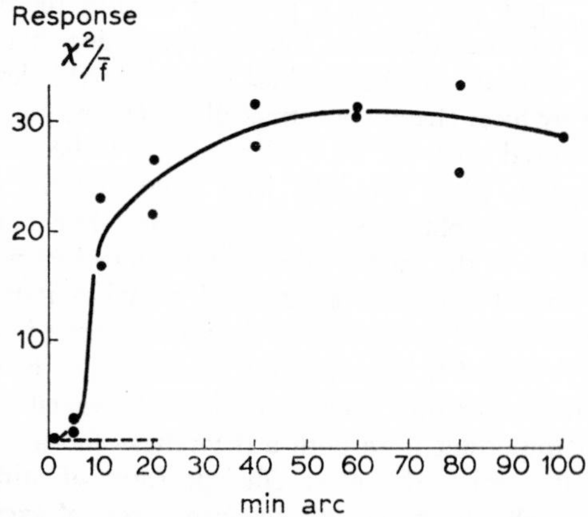

FIG. 37. Responses (ordinate) of a cortical neurone to retinal excitation by horizontal light–dark boundary oscillating at 2 c/s and various amplitudes (abscissa). Interrupted line shows χ^2/f for a stationary border.
(From Burns, Heron & Pritchard, 1962, *J. Neurophysiol.*, **25**, 165, Fig. 8.)

Like cells of the visual cortex, neurones in the auditory cortex seem to respond best to changing environmental conditions. Evans, Ross & Whitfield (1965) found that among 86 neurones responding to sound in the auditory cortex of the unanaesthetized cat, some 35% (30 cells) would only respond at the ON or OFF of an auditory stimulus, or to a note of sliding pitch. The remaining units were classified as giving a 'sustained response' to a steady tone, consisting in either maintained inhibition or excitation of spontaneous activity. It is, however, uncertain for how long this response would have been maintained, since their records show the steady stimulus as lasting only for a second or two.

In somato-sensory cortex of the lightly anaesthetized cat, Mountcastle (1957) has found cells which respond to pressure on the skin by a relatively well-maintained increase in frequency of discharge. Units that were responsive to joint movement also continued to discharge when the relevant joint was held in a steady position. As would be expected, units that could be excited by the movement of hairs adapted rapidly to maintained deflection of hair.

In conclusion, one has to admit that so little is known of cortical function, that generalizations are hard to formulate and have no greater value than that of working hypotheses. It appears at present as though those units that make up the dense felt-work of neurones defined as sensory cortex by classical methods, are more likely to respond to changes than to steady states of the animal's environment. They appear to register local excitation of the cortical network rather than diffuse excitation; they respond better to a train of incoming action potentials than they do to individual signals.

Spatial representation of the environment

The older studies of neuro-anatomy, neurology and physiology have shown that the most used sensory inputs receive the greatest cortical representation. Thus, the central part of the retina, or the forefinger and thumb of the primate, project upon a disproportionately large area of the relevant sensory cortex. It is not clear, however, to what extents constant usage or an inborn distribution of cortical afferents contribute towards the disproportionate representation of most used parts. It can be explained by assuming that a constant quota of cortical representation is allocated to each and every peripheral sensory nerve fibre. The density of sensory fibres to the skin of the forefinger, lips and tongue is far higher than is that for the skin of the back (see Ruch, 1961); the number of optic nerve fibres carrying information from a unit retinal area decreases rapidly as one passes from centre to the periphery (Weymouth, 1958). Daniel & Whitteridge (1961) have shown for the anaesthetized monkey that 1 mm of cortex represents a 6° angle of foveal vision—a cortical magnification factor of 6·0; for vision 15° out from the fovea, 1 mm cortex represents a visual angle of only 0·5°; at 60° from the fovea, the corresponding cortical magnification factor is 0·1. Thus, as one passes from central to peripheral vision, the area of visual cortex representing unit area of retina declines by a factor of some 3600 ($=60^2$). Unfortunately, it is not possible to determine whether each retinal ganglion cell receives an identical allocation of cortical representation, since sufficiently reliable ganglion cell counts are not available. On the other hand, there is good reason to expect a close correspondence between the local density of ganglion cells and the minimum angle of resolution. For the human, both fall off linearly with eccentricity for the first 30° of peripheral vision (Weymouth, 1958). It is therefore interesting that Daniel & Whitteridge found a close correspondence between the reciprocal of cortical magnification factor in the monkey and Weymouth's minimum angle of resolution for man, over some 65° of peripheral vision. These results certainly support the hypothesis that every peripheral sensory fibre receives the same measure of cortical representation.

Thus, the impression that the most used parts of the body receive the greatest cortical representation is partly explained by the fact that the most used parts are most densely innervated by peripheral sensory fibres. On the other hand, this is probably not the whole story; present evidence suggests that cortical 'plasticity' will also contribute to the same end result. Experiments involving the removal of small areas of cortex have suggested that one region of sensory-motor cortex can adopt the functions of a neighbouring damaged area (Glees & Cole, 1950). Wiesel & Hubel have shown (1963) that absence of pattern vision in one eye of kittens leads, after a few months, to a functional disconnection of that retina from neurones in the cerebral cortex. In contrast, three months of monocular deprivation in the adult animal, by lid-closure, resulted in no detectable physiological abnormality.

It could be said that each classical sensory area of the cortex provides a map, on a roughly linear scale, of peripheral afferent nerve fibres. It is, however, a map which indicates more than the location of peripheral input; it shows both the site and type of sensory excitation. A better analogy would be to picture sensory cortex as similar to a map constructed in mosaic, where each stone of the total pattern would indicate the site of excitation by its approximate position, and the nature of excitation by its colour. Mountcastle (1957) has found that all of the neurones encountered by an extracellular micro-electrode, inserted perpendicular to the cortical surface, were excited by the same type of sensory input. Thus, one small column of cells, extending right through the cortical grey matter, would be excited by the movement of hairs in the appropriate part of the periphery; a neighbouring column of cells was excitable by skin pressure in the peripheral district; while disturbance of the deep fascia or joint surfaces of the same region would drive cells of a separate, nearby column. This mosaic-like arrangement of modalities of sensation appears to obtain in the sensory-motor cortex of both cat and monkey (Mountcastle, 1957; Powell & Mountcastle, 1959).

A similar spatial organization of types of sensation has been demonstrated in the visual cortex of both cat and ape (Hubel & Wiesel, 1962, 1963*a*). I have already referred to the fact that cells in the visual cortex are best excited by lines or light–dark borders in the visual field, with a particular orientation. Hubel and Wiesel also found that the cortex was ". . . divisible into discrete columns; within each column the cells all had the same receptive-field axis orientation. The columns appeared to extend from surface to white matter; cross-sectional diameters at the surface were of the order of 0·5 mm." (Fig. 38). Again, one must picture the visual cortex as providing a map in mosaic where each unit of the total pattern is a small column of cells, the disturbance of which indicates for the rest of the nervous system the site and nature of visual excitation.

There is at present no evidence suggesting a similar arrangement of units within the auditory cortex. There is some reason to believe that, on a gross scale, peripheral nerve fibres are mapped spatially across the auditory cortex. For instance, Tunturi (1950) found evidence of such an arrangement in anaesthetized dogs when strychnine was applied to the cortical surface. He observed the potentials evoked by pure tones of threshold loudness and concluded that "The fibres for each frequency terminate in a band no wider than 0·2 mm and 5 to 7 mm in length, extending transversely across the gyrus. In the anterior-posterior direction the bands are arranged as a series of parallel strips with a spacing of 2 mm per octave over the frequency range between 240 and 8000 c.p.s. . . . the low frequencies posteriorly." Evans, Ross & Whitfield (1965) have explored the auditory cortex of the unrestrained, unanaesthetized cat with extracellular micro-electrodes (as opposed to the gross surface electrodes employed by Tunturi) and can find no convincing evidence of tonotopic organization. Nor could they find evidence of a mosaic-like arrangement of cell columns, each peculiarly sensitive to one class of auditory stimulus. It should be noticed, however, that their animals were unanaesthetized and unrestrained and it seems possible that preparations of this sort are not suitable for localization tests. One imagines that anaesthetic, by interfering with multisynaptic conduction, makes the relatively direct pathways more apparent; this certainly seems to be the case when records of evoked potentials are obtained with gross surface electrodes.

In somato-sensory and visual cortex, the evidence for a point-to-point representation of peripheral sensory events seems conclusive; it

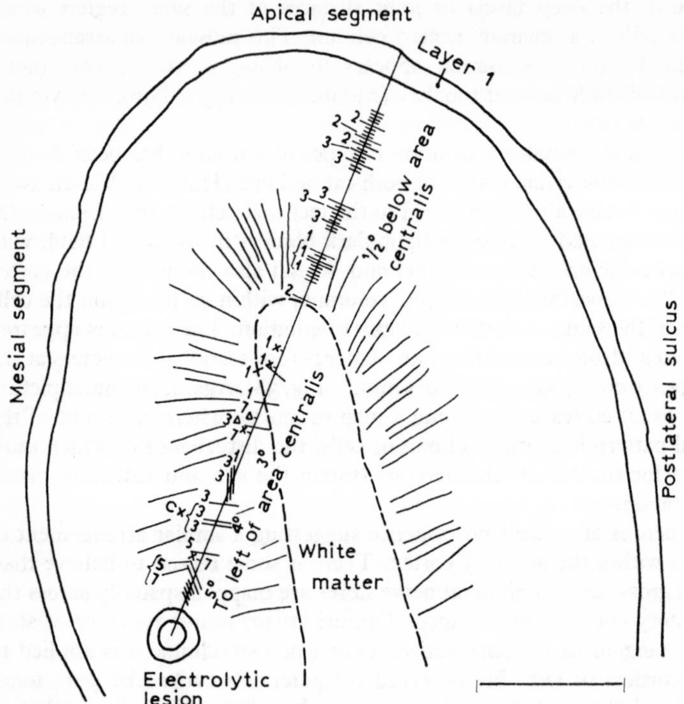

FIG. 38. Reconstruction of micro-electrode penetration through the lateral gyrus. Electrode entered apical segment normal to the surface, and remained parallel to the deep fibre bundles (indicated by radial lines) until reaching white matter; in grey matter of mesial segment the electrode's course was oblique. Longer lines represent cortical cells. Axons of cortical cells are indicated by a cross-bar at right-hand end of line. Field-axis orientation is shown by the direction of each line; lines perpendicular to track represent vertical orientation. Brace-brackets show simultaneously recorded units. Complex receptive fields are indicated by 'Cx'. Afferent fibres from the lateral geniculate body indicated by X, for ON centre; Δ, for OFF centre. Approximate positions of receptive fields on the retina are shown to the right of the penetration. Shorter lines show regions in which unresolved background activity was observed. Scale = 1 mm.
(From Hubel & Wiesel, 1962, *J. Physiol.*, **160,** 106, Fig. 13.)

implies a relatively direct and dense anatomical pathway between particular peripheral sensory nerve fibres and their 'representative' cortical neurones. It does not, of course, follow that the response of cortical cells provides a faithful map of the spatial distribution of external events. A white triangle in the visual field will produce a similar triangular patch of light upon the retina, and the consequent excitation of ganglion cells must produce a spatial pattern of excited neurones in the visual cortex, which has some triangular characteristics.

Linear distortion of the cortical analogue will be introduced by the variable neural magnification factor referred to above. Moreover, there is no reason to presume that this pattern would excite all of the cortical units within a triangular area of the visual cortex. In fact, the observation that cortical neurones will only respond to local changes of retinal illumination, suggests that a visual target of this sort should produce three lines of excited units, representing only the borders of the solid triangular figure in the visual field. The involuntary movements of physiological nystagmus would ensure that the borders of the visual target caused a continual local fluctuation of illumination restricted to three straight lines within the retina. These considerations, and also the existence of lateral inhibition in both retina and lateral geniculate body, suggest that patterns of excitation in the visual cortex should bear some close relation to the first differential of light intensity across the visual field.

This was found to be the case by Burns, Heron & Pritchard (1962) who examined the responses of cortical neurones in the isolated forebrain of the unanaesthetized cat. They recorded post-stimulus histograms obtained from single cells in the visual cortex responding to artificial saccadic movements of simple patterns in the visual field. The patterns used were focused upon one retina with a spectacle lens; the other eye received no light. Responses were tested to a single, straight, black–white border at a number of different positions in the visual field; the orientation of the border was always the same and was near to the optimum for the cell in question. It was found that there was only one position of the pattern giving a maximal response, while the magnitude of the evoked response fell off steeply as the pattern was displaced from this position (Fig. 39). If the pattern was rotated to a new orientation and the process repeated, another maximal position could be found. The point of intersection of the two borders providing maximal responses could be said to lie within a *representative district* for the recorded unit—a district of the visual field, within which movement of any border is most likely to produce a response. Burns & Pritchard (1964) described such tests as determining a 'representative point', which is a somewhat misleading nomenclature, since subsequent results have shown that the exact position of a pattern eliciting maximal unit response is often influenced by the precise manner of pattern exposure. The results of Fig. 39 suggest that the response of a cortical unit depends upon the proximity of its representative district to any neighbouring intensity gradients in the visual field. It should follow that the cortical excitation of a cell whose representative district lies at the centre of any small pattern of light, is greater than that produced by a similar but larger pattern of light. Figure 40 shows that this is the case for two squares of light presented upon a black background.

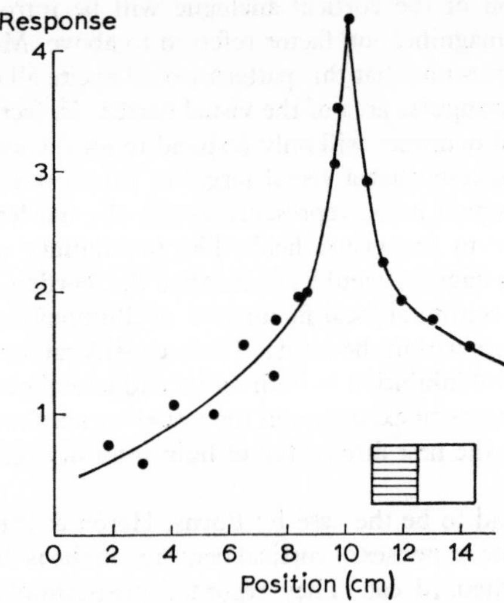

FIG. 39. The variation of unit response with position of a light–dark border in the visual field. Derived from records of the discharge of a neurone in the visual cortex (cat's unanaesthetized, isolated forebrain) during excitation of the contralateral retina with a border given artificial saccades of amplitude 50 min arc at 1 c/s. Ordinate = peak response in post-stimulus histogram; arbitrary units. Abscissa = position of border on ground-glass screen; 1 cm represents 1° 24′ at the retina.

Figure 39 makes it clear that a straight edge oscillating at one point in the visual field must set up a relatively widespread excitation of cells within the visual cortex. Mandl (personal communication) has shown that 1° of central vision in the cat is represented by some 2 mm across the cortex; thus, the straight edge of Fig. 39 must have modified the behaviour of cells over a strip of visual cortex at least 12 mm wide. Unfortunately, one cannot easily record by a direct method the spread of unit excitation produced by simple patterns; it is not possible to record responses to a fixed pattern position from a series of functionally similar units at various cortical sites. On the other hand, one can assume that the unit of Fig. 39 is one member of a large population of similar cells, spread with even density across the cortex in a tangential layer. Figure 39 could then be regarded as indicating the spatial distribution of excitation across the cortex for this particular cell type.

The results discussed above suggest that the brain might record a pattern in the visual field as the locations of a series of intensity gradients, each indicated by a group of particularly active cortical units. However, inspection of Fig. 41 shows clearly that positions of maximal activity in the visual cortex do not provide an unambiguous index of

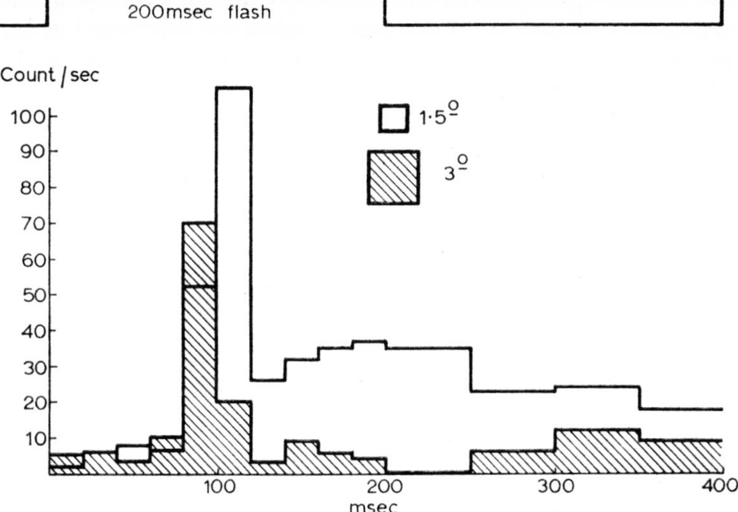

FIG. 40. The responses of a cortical unit to a 1·5° square of light and to a 3° square of light. The representative district for the neurone lay at the centre of these squares.

(Burns & Heron, unpublished data.)

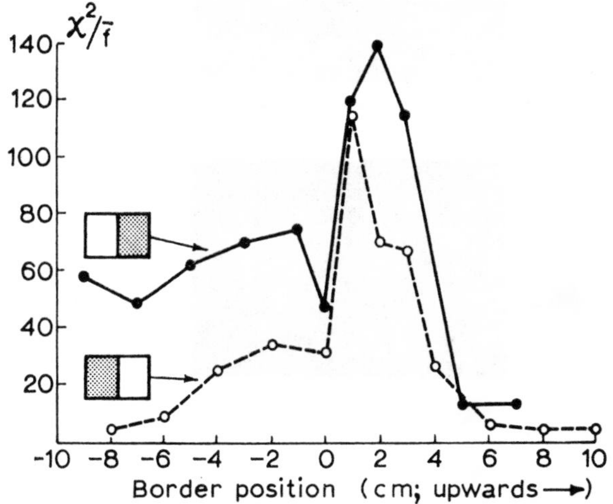

FIG. 41. Variation of the response of a visual neurone with variation of the position of a straight black–white border in the visual field. The pattern was given a rectangular, cyclical oscillation of about 0·5° amplitude at 3 c/s for 2 min. Ordinate: response, determined from the post-stimulus histogram as χ^2/mean frequency (Burns, Heron & Pritchard, 1962). Abscissa: position of edge in visual field; 1 cm = 1°.

(From Burns & Pritchard, 1964, *J. Physiol.*, **175**, 445, Fig. 1.)

the positions of borders in the visual field. In this experiment, the approximate cortical site of maximal excitation was determined by the position of the light–dark border in the field; but reversal of the straight-edged pattern (rotation through 180°) shifted the representative position by 1°. Mandl (1968) has shown that, if peak excitation in the post-stimulus histogram is taken as a measure of response, the representative position providing greatest response to a single, straight light–dark border is influenced by:

1. the orientation of the pattern (as in Fig. 41),
2. the method of retinal excitation; flashing or artificial saccadic movements.

Observations such as these make Burns and Pritchard's use of the term 'representative point' meaningless. It becomes clear that there is

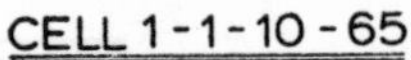

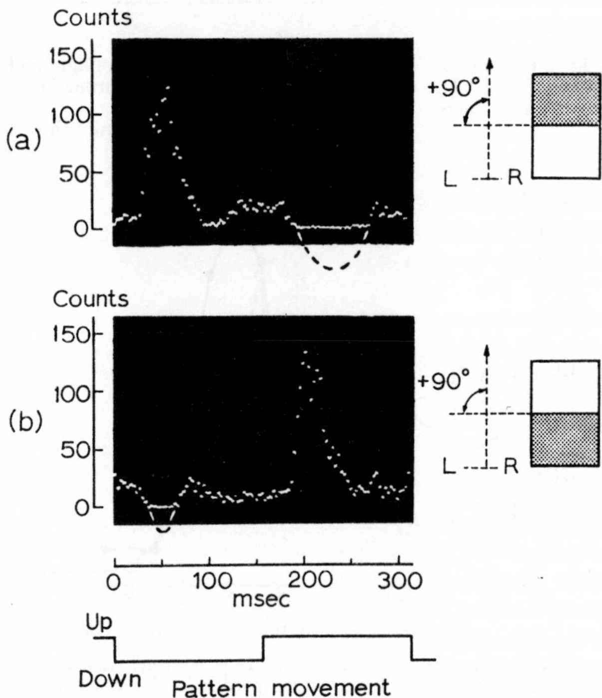

FIG. 42. Post-stimulus histograms from a neurone exhibiting both positive and negative responses to a light–dark border. The interrupted lines below the abscissa were drawn by eye.
(From Mandl, 1968, in preparation.)

no one point in the visual field through which a border must always pass in order to produce maximal unit excitation. It also follows that the location of maximal activity in the visual cortex cannot be the criterion used by the nervous system to identify the position of patterns in the visual field.

It now appears that Burns & Pritchard (1964) were misled by measuring only excitatory cortical responses to retinal excitation; they failed to observe that movement of a pattern in the visual field is almost as likely to produce inhibition of cortical units as it is to excite them. Since the word 'inhibition' has recently acquired the status of a technical term, it would perhaps be safe to refer to the 'negative response' of cortical neurones as opposed to their positive or excitatory response. The behaviour of a visual unit giving a negative response to one direction of pattern movement is illustrated in Fig. 42*a*; reversal of the pattern by rotation through 180°, without change in position of the light–dark border, reversed the behaviour of the cell so that the negative response of Fig. 42*a* became a positive response to the same direction of pattern movement (Fig. 42*b*). It will be seen that pattern reversal also altered the excitatory response of Fig. 42*a* to a negative response of similar latency in Fig. 42*b*. This phenomenon is commonly encountered. The negative response usually appears in the post-stimulus histogram as a period of complete inactivity. Thus, while it is always easy to measure its duration, it is often difficult or impossible to assess its magnitude accurately. The size of a relatively weak negative response can sometimes be measured by artificially increasing the overall mean firing rate of the recorded unit. This can be done by illuminating the visual field of either eye with light flashes which are not 'locked' in any way to the cyclical movements of the test pattern. The results of this manœuvre are illustrated in Fig. 43. But even this procedure usually fails to produce measurable firing during the period of negative response and, more often than not, one is forced to estimate the magnitude of negative responses by eye, in the crude manner illustrated by the interrupted lines of Fig. 42.

When both positive and negative responses to pattern movement are taken into account, cells of the visual cortex yield an astonishing variety of relations between response and position of border in the visual field. The forms of position plot encountered among 33 units in the unanaesthetized cat are illustrated schematically in Fig. 44, parts *a* and *c*. Mandl (1968), like Hubel & Wiesel (1962), suggests that the type of position plot obtained from a visual neurone depends upon the number and type of retinal ganglion cells with which it is closely connected. He concludes that the number of ganglion cells which can influence the behaviour of a cortical unit in this sort of experiment is small and probably not more than three. An illustration of this way of thinking is

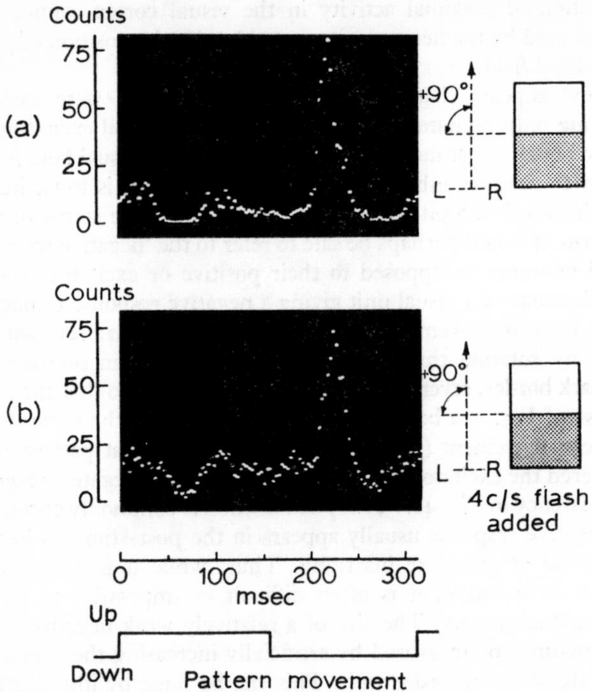

FIG. 43. Post-stimulus histograms from a cell excited by a light–dark oscillating border. Amplitude of border movement = 0·15°. White part of pattern = approx. 5 millilamberts. (*a*) No background excitation. (*b*) Same stimulus with a background flash added at 4 c/s. Intensity of flash = 3 millilamberts.
(From Mandl, 1968, in preparation.)

provided in Fig. 44*b*, which shows the circular, central fields of retinal ganglion cells controlling activity of the corresponding cortical units of Fig. 44*a*, immediately above. An unshaded circle in Fig. 44*b*, indicates the field of a ganglion cell that is excited by increasing illumination and inhibited by decrease of light. Likewise, a shaded circle indicates the field of a ganglion cell with the complementary properties.

The system of connections illustrated by Fig. 44*b* is unrealistically simple, yet is sufficient to indicate the way in which connection with a few ganglion cells might explain the responses of Fig. 44*a*, representing some 75% of cortical units. The properties of the remaining 25% of cortical neurones, illustrated in Fig. 44*c*, could not be explained in the same manner. In any case, the retinal fields of ganglion cells are not as

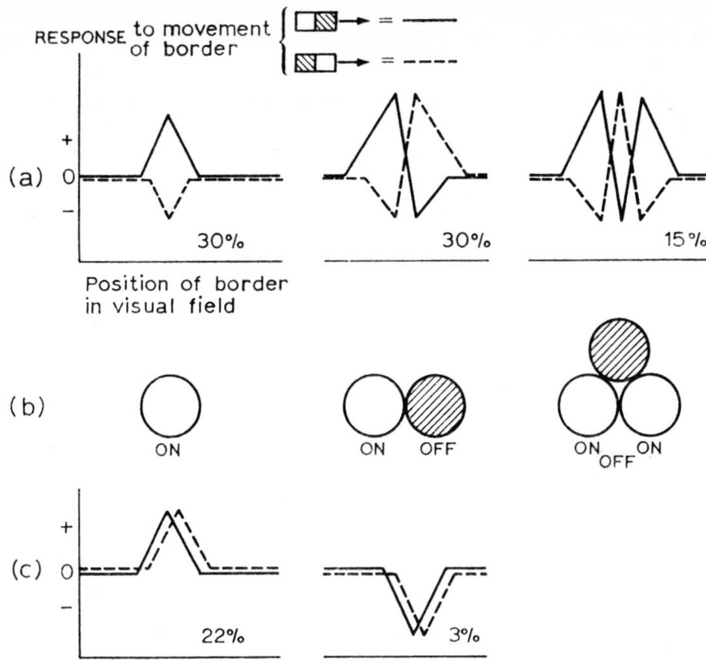

FIG. 44

(*a*) and (*c*) show the various forms of position plot obtained from visual neurones, together with the approximate frequencies with which they are encountered.

(*b*) Combinations of the receptive fields of retinal ganglion cells which might explain the position plots in (*a*). (See text.)
(After Mandl, 1968, in preparation.)

simple as implied by the circles of Fig. 44*b*, which ignores the antagonistic surrounds. Moreover, recent evidence (Spinelli, 1966) suggests that the fields of ganglion cells in the unanaesthetized cat are not always circular, as originally suggested by Kuffler (1953).

The diversity of position plots encountered in the visual cortex makes it unlikely that there is any one aspect of the behaviour of all visual neurones which can serve as an indication of pattern position. The small saccadic movement of a pattern's edge across the retina will excite some visual units and inhibit others. Consequently, the movement of this edge will define a narrow band of visual cortex, within which neighbouring units must display a great difference of instantaneous discharge rates. Mandl (1968) estimates that of every 10 cortical nerve cells responding to the movement of a border in the visual field, roughly 4 will give a negative response, while 6 will respond with a transient increase of firing rate. Thus, the code used by the visual cortex for transmitting information to the rest of the nervous system concerning the position of light–dark borders on the retina is in terms of the relative behaviour of neighbouring neurones or groups of neurones. A bright point-source of light in the visual field will be recorded by the brain as a small district of the visual cortex, within which neighbouring units are discharging at very different rates; when some are firing in excess of their resting frequency, the frequency of others will be diminished.

Temporal representation of the environment

The mosaic-like map of sensory projection upon the cerebral cortex implies that some change in the behaviour of neurones in sensory cortex will indicate to the rest of the brain the presence of a particular class and site of peripheral excitation. While the experiments discussed above describe some of the ways in which sensory excitation can alter the behaviour of cortical neurones, they do not indicate which aspects of the evoked response are of physiological importance. One would like to know the code by which one neurone or group of neurones communicates with another.

The problem is very well illustrated by reference to visual contrast discrimination. Curves of the sort provided in Figs. 39 and 41 suggest that the distribution of excitation across the cortex, produced by a small artificial saccadic movement given to a black–white edge, is often more or less symmetrical about a peak. Taken at its face value, this observation would imply that a cat could not tell the difference between a black mouse on a white background and a white mouse against a dark background. This seems unlikely! It is more probable that responses estimated from the post-stimulus histogram (as peak height or χ^2) do not describe the aspect of neuronal behaviour which is important to this form of discrimination by the intact animal.

Burns & Pritchard (1964) investigated the problem of contrast discrimination, using essentially the same techniques that have been described above. After the tip of the recording micropipette had been lodged next to a cortical neurone, the representative district for this neurone was determined. Records were then obtained of the cell's response to artificial saccadic movements of a straight, light–dark edge, oscillating in the vicinity of the representative district. The object of these experiments was to investigate the difference in behaviour of a neurone representing first the light side and then the dark side of the border. Consequently, the first test would be run with the exciting border oscillating about a mean position that was a degree or so away from the centre of the representative district; the amplitude of saccadic movements was never such as to carry the edge across this central point. During the first test, the centre of the representative district might be on the light side of the light–dark boundary. The next test would then be made with the centre of the representative district on the dark side of the boundary and at the same distance from it; this was effected either by rotating the pattern through 180°, or by moving the edge to the other side of the representative district, without change in its orientation (Fig. 45).

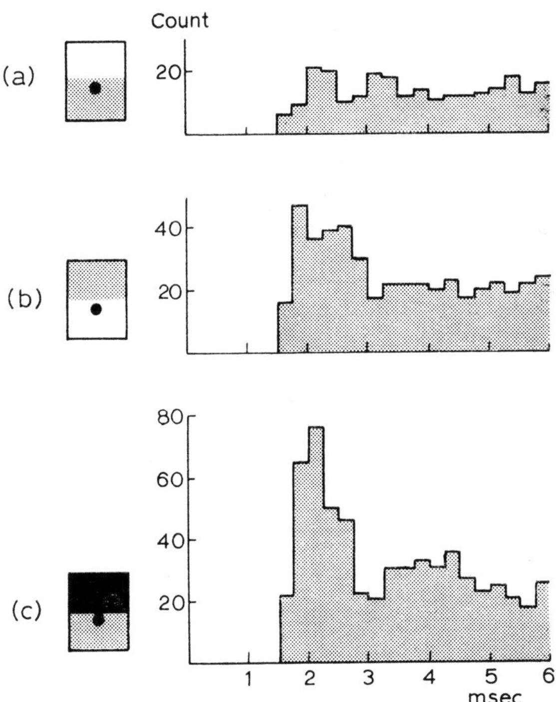

FIG. 45. Autocorrelograms from a visual neurone excited by grey–white and black–grey borders. In all cases the representative point for the unit was 0·5° from the border. In (*a*) this point was on the grey side of the border; in (*b*) it was on the white side of the grey–white border used. In (*c*) this point was on the grey side of the black–grey border.
(From Burns & Pritchard, 1964, *J. Physiol.*, **175**, 445, Fig. 6.)

There appeared to be four ways in which the behaviour of cells might differ when representing the light and dark sides of a boundary. The behaviour of 8 cells tested in 7 cats exposed to an oscillating black–white boundary could be classified as follows:

a. Three cells provided post-stimulus histograms which showed several peaks following each direction of pattern movement whenever the cell was representing the dark part of the visual field; when representing the light part of the field, these cells showed only one peak after movement of the pattern.

b. Five cells gave a more pronounced response (in the post-stimulus histogram) to one direction of pattern movement than the other (Fig. 21). The most stimulating direction of pattern movement depended upon whether these units were representing the light or dark sides of the boundary; but whether representation of light or dark provided the greatest response, varied from unit to unit.

c. Four cells representing the light parts of the visual field provided autocorrelograms displaying a much more regular rhythm than did the autocorrelograms from the same cells when representing the dark part of the field.

d. All 8 of these cells discharged with a larger number of short intervals between action potentials when representing the light part of the visual field than they did when representing the dark side of the boundary (Figs. 26 and 45).

It was shown that the behaviour of neurones as classified above was not dependent upon the absolute light intensity to which their representative districts were exposed. The nature of their response appeared to be governed only by the direction of the gradient of light intensity across any border near to the representative district (Fig. 45). It was not apparently dependent upon the form of pattern employed as a stimulus, since tests with circular patterns and two-edged bars produced essentially the same results. When the results were pooled from experiments in which a variety of patterns and light-intensity gradients were used, it was found that the frequencies of behaviour of the types listed above were distributed as follows:

Class of behaviour	*a*	*b*	*c*	*d*
% of 21 tests on 10 neurones in 9 cats	43	62	48	100

It is possible that any or all of the differences in behaviour listed above may form the basis of a code by which the intact animal discriminates light from relative darkness in the visual field. There may be certain cells that are reserved for relaying this sort of information to the rest of the nervous system; or, alternatively, contrast discrimination may depend upon a behavioural code that is common to all neurones of the visual cortex. Codes *a*, *b* and *c* are only operated by some of the neurones in the visual cortex and could indicate the existence of specialized units for contrast discrimination. However, codes *a* and *b* describe responses in terms of peaks in the post-stimulus histogram and it does not seem very likely that such criteria could form the basis of contrast discrimination. A post-stimulus histogram can only be constructed from a knowledge of the times and directions of pattern movements used in the experiments. For the nervous system of the intact animal to perform a similar analysis, information concerning local changes in retinal illumination would have to be cross-correlated with the times and directions of involuntary eye movements. However, present evidence suggests that information about eye movements is not fed back to higher levels within the nervous system (Brindley & Merton, 1960). The behaviour described under *c* above undoubtedly requires the presence of repeated cyclic movements of the exciting pattern across the retina, and because the movements of physiological nystagmus are never of this nature (Ratliff & Riggs, 1950; Ditchburn & Ginsborg, 1953), the experimental observations are not directly relevant to normal contrast discrimination.

The only class of behaviour identified by Burns and Pritchard which remains as a candidate for the basis of contrast discrimination is class *d* which was exhibited by all of the small number of visual neurones which they held for long enough to expose to a variety of tests. This suggests that all units in the visual cortex may be capable of generating the signals necessary to recognition of the light and relatively dark parts of a visual field. Such identification by the rest of the nervous system would depend upon the fact that visual units representing the brighter side of boundaries in the exciting pattern discharged with a greater number of short intervals between their action potentials than did similar neighbours representing the other, darker, sides of these boundaries. If this is, in fact, the code used by the nervous system for contrast discrimination, it is not hard to visualize the way in which other central neurones might make use of the information. No function more complex than temporal summation would be required of an 'observer cell', which would then fire only when receiving from neurones representing the relatively bright side of a boundary near to their representative district.

Universal and specific codes

The finding that all of a small number of neurones in the visual cortex have provided a code of behaviour which would enable an observer to decide whether they were representing the light or relatively dark parts of a pattern in the visual field, does not prove that contrast discrimination depends upon this type of behaviour. It merely offers one physiological mechanism upon which such discrimination by the normal animal *might* depend; and suggests, moreover, that all units of the visual cortex may be capable of relaying the relevant information. It is not impossible that contrast discrimination depends, in fact, upon some other form of signal that is transmitted by only a few specialized cells. Hubel & Wiesel (1962) have demonstrated the existence of neurones capable of doing this job. In the cat there are some units exhibiting what they have called 'simple cortical receptive fields', that respond best when excited by a light–dark boundary presented in the appropriate part of the visual field with a specific orientation (Fig. 46).

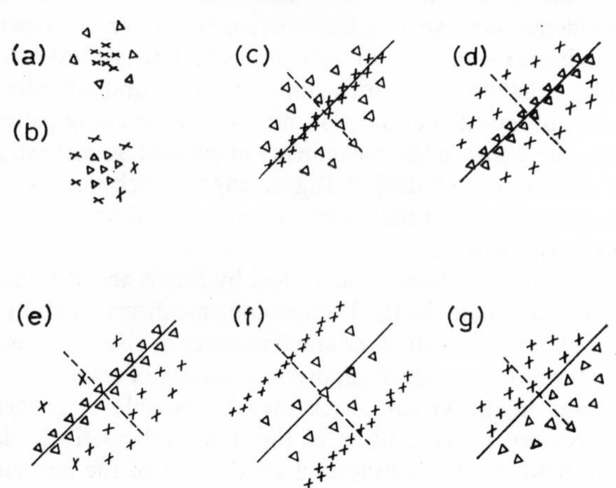

FIG. 46. Common arrangements of lateral geniculate and cortical receptive fields.

(*a*) ON centre geniculate receptive field.

(*b*) OFF centre geniculate receptive field.

(*c–g*) Various arrangements of simple cortical receptive fields. X, areas giving excitatory responses (ON responses); Δ, areas giving inhibitory responses (OFF responses). Receptive field axes are shown by continuous lines through field centres; in the figure these are all oblique, but each arrangement occurs in all orientations.

(From Hubel & Wiesel, 1962, *J. Physiol.*, **160,** 106, Fig. 2.)

Some patterns in the visual field could be unambiguously described by the response of such units alone. For instance, a single straight light–dark border, extending right across the visual field, is a pattern that will display a single orientation. A black triangle upon a white background (Fig. 47*a*) provides only three orientations of light–dark border, but is not the only simple pattern with this property, as can be seen from Fig. 47*b*. To define a pattern with the shape in Fig. 47*a*, one must specify also the orientation of one of the angles of the triangle; the junctions between *A*- and *B*-type receptors must be described as relatively light on the convex side. It is therefore interesting that Hubel and Wiesel have found angle detectors in the cat (Fig. 70, Chapter 7); these appear to be visual units which will only respond when a particular angle of light–dark border is presented with a specific orientation in the visual field. Another way in which the two triangles of Fig. 47 might be

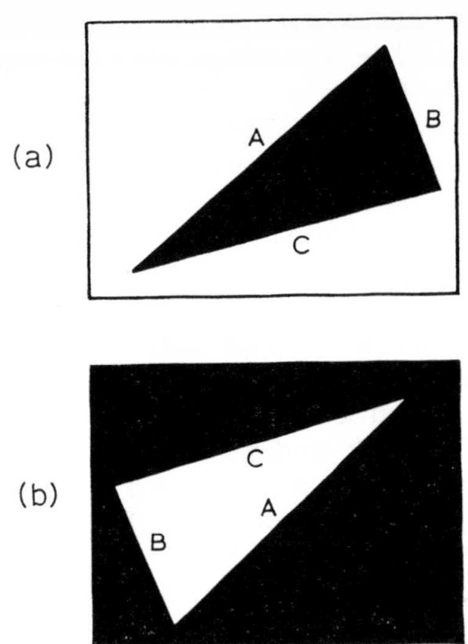

FIG. 47. Two different figures providing the same orientations of light–dark border.

distinguished by the nervous system could depend upon Burns and Pritchard's observation that neurones representing the darker parts of a visual field fire with relatively few short intervals between spikes.

Experiments designed to record the statistical behaviour of neurones in the visual cortex have produced no results that are inconsistent with Hubel and Wiesel's observations. They merely stress another aspect of cell function. Where Hubel and Wiesel's experiments with lightly anaesthetized animals have been designed to detect the specific differences of behaviour between cells, the statistical analysis of records from unanaesthetized cortex was intended to demonstrate those universal properties that were common to all visual units. Hubel & Wiesel (1962) found no indication from their studies that the striate cortex contained nerve cells which were unresponsive to visual stimuli, but some of their units could only be excited by stimuli with very specific properties. The behaviour of cells with 'complex receptive fields' could not be predicted from tests with small flashing light-spots; they responded to such stimuli as the movement of light–dark edges of proper orientation anywhere within the visual field. The results of statistical experiments with unanaesthetized cortex, excited by larger patterns in the visual field, provide a different impression of cell specificity. Examined in this way, visual units appear to be slightly less fussy about the type of stimulus required to drive them. Under these conditions, any cell appears to respond to some extent to the saccadic movement of any pattern within a few degrees of its representative district. But, in agreement with Hubel and Wiesel's findings, every cell responds best when the edge crosses the field at a specific angle and passes through a particular representative district. The different pictures of cell behaviour provided by the two techniques are slight, but may be important.

In any case, both sets of observation stress the importance of orientation of exciting pattern. The fact that each column of cells in the mosaic of columns forming the visual cortex requires a specific orientation of border for its optimal excitation, may explain why the nervous system is so much better at the identification of shape, than of size or position of pattern in the visual field. The details of pattern perception may depend upon the activity of cortical units, specifically reserved for the detection of light–dark borders, angles and movement as Hubel and Wiesel's results imply. It is a little hard to believe, however, that every small region of cortex contains sufficient angle detectors to represent all recognizable angles and all possible orientations of angle. Alternatively, some of the specificity that their experiments have undoubtedly revealed may be the consequence of fortuitous connections among a population of orientation-sensitive units.

Optical illusions

Several forms of neural behaviour have been discussed above, which could represent the essential physiological codes by which the normal intact animal identifies the positions of borders in the visual field, or distinguishes the light from darker areas in that field. The type of experiment from which this information is derived does not allow one to determine whether a code which transmits the information necessary to a particular form of discrimination is, in fact, used. It seems that this can only be decided by behavioural studies in the intact animal; one needs to know whether these temporal patterns of neural discharge are always associated with responses based upon the form of sensory discrimination in question. Alternatively, and this is often technically easier, it may be possible to predict that confusion of interpretation will occur in certain circumstances, if a particular code of neural behaviour does form the basis of normal perception. Thus, when considering the behaviour of neurones in the visual cortex, any code which is successful in predicting optical illusions is likely to be of physiological importance.

This point is illustrated by the following discussion of some well-known optical illusions. The so-called Müller–Lyer illusion (Fig. 48*a*) appears to be entirely consistent with neurophysiological data suggesting that all cortical units are orientation-specific. The upper horizontal line of Fig. 48*a* seems longer than the lower horizontal line, although this is not the case. The expected cortical distribution of neurones, maximally excited by these two patterns in the visual field, is shown in

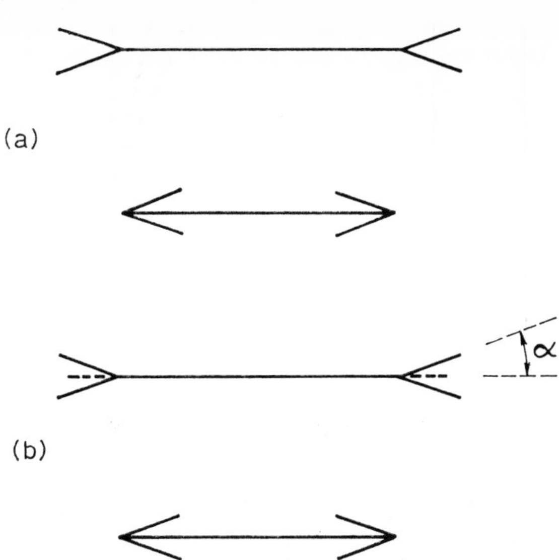

FIG. 48. Illustrating the Müller–Lyer illusion. (See text.)

Fig. 48*b*. The dotted lines indicate units that are strongly excited by the horizontal component of both neighbouring divergent lines in the upper figure, and would be responsible for the nervous system's interpreting the upper horizontal line as longer. This would be the expected result of the orientation-specificity of visual neurones. Those neurones lying along the dotted lines of Fig. 48*b* should be excited by a component from both diverging lines in the visual field, proportional to cosine α. Heymans found (1896) that the magnitude of the Müller–Lyer illusion was, in fact, proportional to cos α.

There is another well-known optical illusion which is worth matching against physiological expectation. The two broad lines of Fig. 49*a* are in fact parallel, although they appear to diverge at the upper ends. Now, Hubel and Wiesel's results have stressed the importance of orientation of light–dark edges in the visual field, and suggest that complex patterns might be recorded by the brain, primarily in terms of the local orientations of their borders. There seems little doubt that the majority, if not all, of the units in the cat's visual cortex are orientation-specific. The question is whether this specificity forms an essential part of the neural code in which the information necessary to perception is transmitted; is a pattern identified by the nervous system's asking, "Which class of orientation receptors were excited in each part of the visual system?" If this were so, we should expect that the right-hand side of the pattern in Fig. 49*a* would produce large responses from two

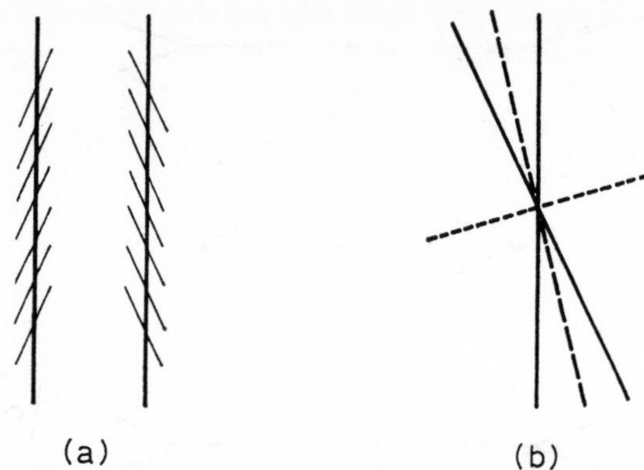

FIG. 49. Illustrating the apparent divergence of parallel lines, produced by superimposition of a herring-bone pattern. (See text.)

classes of orientation-specific visual unit—those units sensitive to the orientations illustrated with continuous lines in Fig. 49*b*. Each of these two primary orientations on the right-hand side of Fig. 49*a* would produce some excitation of units that were optimally excitable by other orientations of pattern. The response of these units (in fact, of all units) should be proportional to the cosine of the angle between their specific orientation and actual orientation of the exciting border. Thus, one would expect a maximal 'secondary excitation' of units specifically sensitive to the interrupted lines of Fig. 49*b*. These represent orientations maximally excitable by the sum of the two primary orientations. One would expect units with an orientation-specificity indicated by the dashed line to be more excited than those excited by the dotted line, which bisects the greater angle between lines in the original figure. Thus, according to this way of thinking, the pattern of Fig. 49*a* should produce a maximal excitation of units specifically sensitive to orientations bisecting the acute angles between the thick and thin intersecting lines of Fig. 49*a*. The pattern of Fig. 49*a* should then produce the illusion that the two thick lines converge toward the upper end. In fact this pattern produces just the opposite impression.

This illusion does not appear to be consistent with the assumption that the interpretation of patterns depends upon the orientation sensitivity of cortical units. Unfortunately, no data are available to support a more satisfactory hypothesis.

Of course, an argument of this type cannot prove anything. It merely provides a little support for the following beliefs:

1. that cortical units are orientation-specific, being excited in proportion to the cosine of the angle between an appropriately placed,

light–dark border in the visual field and the direction to which they are most sensitive;
2. that the nervous system does not make direct use of this orientation-specificity when recording the directions of borders in a visual pattern.

The main purpose of the discussion above was to illustrate the manner in which optical illusions can be used for testing hypotheses derived from neurophysiological observation. A similar use is made of optical illusions in that part of Chapter 6 which is concerned with binocular vision.

Teleological approach to the problem of sensory coding

Teleological reasoning is unfashionable. Nevertheless, despite any dangers that accompany this way of thinking, it provides an approach to a complex set of observations that may at least suggest new tests and experiments, and can sometimes sort out likely from less likely hypotheses. Thus, it may be helpful to ask: "How might one build a nervous system, capable of distinguishing different patterns in the visual field?" This, in fact, is a very practical question for those electrical engineers and logicians engaged on the construction of pattern-recognizing inputs to man-made computers. Clearly, the discovery of an elegant and economical solution to this problem of engineering would not prove that the mammalian nervous system operated in a similar manner. (The fact that the wheel provides a simple method of transporting loads does not prove that mammals have wheels!) On the other hand, the same necessity for economy in numbers and types of components will limit the choice of the engineer as it must have limited natural selection; and the probability that both processes will reach similar goals seems high.

The problem, then, is to design a nervous system:

1. that will readily identify shape, despite considerable variation in position, magnitude and orientation in the visual field;
2. that requires the smallest possible total number of parts;
3. belonging to a small number of different functional types; and
4. assembled with a minimum of anatomical organization.

The importance of the first two of these specifications to survival is self-evident; a lion must look like a lion at many ranges and must remain identifiable, whether it is walking up hill or down. At the same time, the weight and volume of the brain required for its recognition must not be so great that escape is impossible. A need for reliability of operation leads to specifications 3 and 4; it is clear that the smaller the number of specifications required to construct an instrument containing a fixed number of components, the smaller will be the chance of failure due to malfunction of one component.

The receptive fields of retinal ganglion cells, which supply the brain with information, have usually been described as circular and of two types—centre ON (with OFF periphery) and centre OFF (with peripheral ON). These fields have been estimated as covering about 20° for peripheral vision in the frog (Barlow, 1953), 6° for central vision in the cat (Kuffler, 1953) and 4′—2° for the monkey (Hubel & Wiesel, 1960). It is convenient for the present argument to simplify the real situation and to consider the central nervous system as supplied by approximately equal numbers of ON- and OFF-type ganglion cells, each responding in the appropriate way to change of illumination within a circle of visual field. In Fig. 50, these receptive fields are illustrated as shaded (= OFF

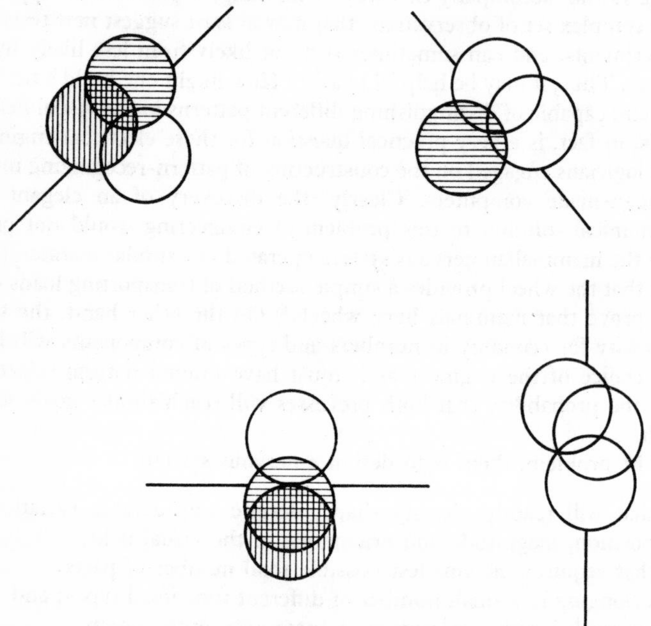

FIG. 50. The formation of orientation-sensitive cortical receptive fields by the random selection of neighbouring retinal receptive fields, taken three at a time. Shaded circles = OFF retinal fields; unshaded circles = ON retinal fields. The straight lines indicate in each case the orientation of a straight, light–dark border that is most likely to excite.

type) and unshaded (= ON type) circles. Hubel and Wiesel have observed that information leaving the retina is altered little by passage through the lateral geniculate body; the receptive fields of geniculate neurones are circular and very similar to those of ganglion cells. In contrast, the receptive fields of units in the visual cortex are elongated; Hubel & Wiesel (1962) have suggested that each cortical neurone is readily excited by a small number of retinal ganglion cells, and that the elongated fields of cortical units are thus built up from the fusion of several of the more peripheral, circular fields. Let us suppose, then, that each cortical neurone is connected at random to excitatory inputs from a small number—say three—of ganglion cells with neighbouring receptive fields. One would then expect to find all cortical units to be more or less orientation-specific, in that a straight line could always be drawn across the retina separating an area that contained mostly ON- from one containing mostly OFF-centre receptive fields. This point is illustrated in Fig. 50. One would expect to find all possible orientations equally represented in the visual cortex; Hubel and Wiesel's careful analysis suggests that this may be so. Moreover, if each cortical neurone were to receive excitation from a small number of optic radiations that ascended radially through the cortical grey matter, one would expect cortical units of similar orientation-specificity to be found in columns. Unfortunately there is little evidence for such a tidy arrangement of the optic radiations. Sholl (1956) describes them as ending in "... up to twelve main branches, the distance between the extreme branches being as much as 650 μ and the terminations occurring at different depths in the main stellate zone". Thus, Hubel & Wiesel (1963*a*) were forced to assume a radial distribution of incoming excitation, without knowledge of any anatomical correlate. The recent observations of Colonnier (1964) may offer the missing structural explanation. The anatomical facts do at least provide a structural basis for the 500 μ diameters of the columns of cells with similar orientation-specificity found by Hubel & Wiesel (1962). In any case, the argument above suggests that the observed orientation-specificity of cortical units may be the accidental result of random connections between optic radiations and the cortical neurones that lie within some 250 μ of their ascending terminals.

An instrument designed to identify the shape of patterns in the visual field, without regard to their position or magnitude, must assess the orientations presented by the light–dark borders of the pattern. This could be done by recording the various classes of orientation-sensitive cortical neurones that were excited by the pattern, in the manner dis-discussed on p. 102. But the construction of such an instrument would require a great number of specified connections. It would necessitate, for instance:

1. that each small cortical district were capable of recording many different orientations of border;
2. that 'observer cells' existed, possibly outside the visual area, for the

purpose of registering the various orientations presented by any pattern;

3. that each of the observer cells for recording the presence of a specific orientation somewhere in the visual field should receive connections from all the appropriate orientation-specific units in the visual cortex.

Many interneuronal connections would be necessary and they would require careful specification.

There is at least one way of constructing an instrument capable of pattern recognition from a smaller number of neural elements, assembled with less rigid specifications. We have already pointed out in Chapter 4 that waves of excitation can spread through a network of

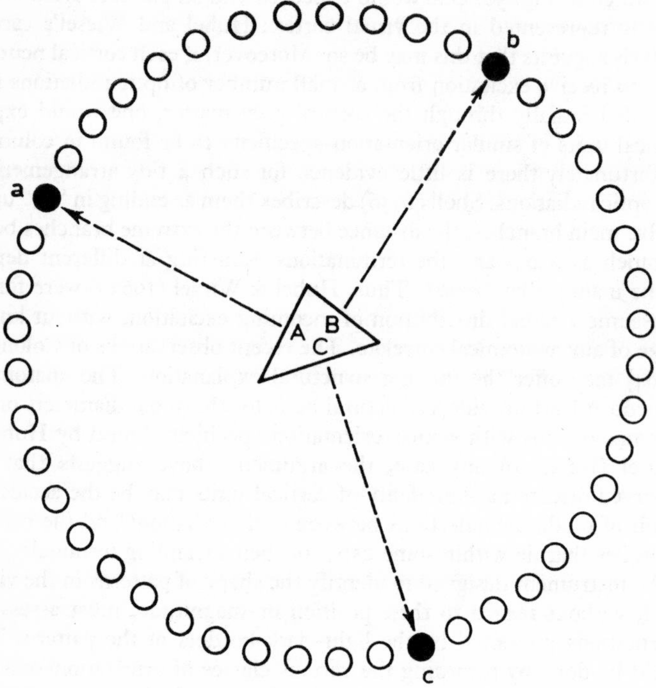

FIG. 51. The operation of a hypothetical plane network of pattern-identifying neurones. (See text.)

randomly interconnected neurones. There is, in fact, evidence that the cortex contains such a network of neurones, spread across the brain's surface. Suppose now that a simple pattern of excitation, such as the triangle of Fig. 51, occurs near the centre of a network of this sort. Waves of excitation will travel outwards across the network, in directions perpendicular to the sides of the triangular focus, in somewhat the same way as waves would spread across the surface of a lake if a triangular form were dropped into it. If the spreading waves attenuate with distance from their points of origin and the propagation velocity were dependent upon their magnitude, as seems likely in intact cortex (Beurle, 1956), then the maximum velocities of transmission will occur along the dotted lines of Fig. 51. Suppose now that the uniform neural net of Fig. 51 were bordered by a ring of 'observer neurones', the postulated triangular focus of excitation would cause the simultaneous excitation of observer units *a*, *b* and *c*. These same observer cells would be excited, whatever the size of the central triangle, and in this way the pattern would be correctly interpreted regardless of its absolute size in the visual field. The addition of another class of observer cells, capable of estimating the distances *ab*, *bc* and *ca*, could provide a system able to identify the form of the central triangle, independent of its magnitude or its orientation.

There is no point in pushing this argument further, since enough has already been said to stress the way in which a teleological approach may be helpful. The description of any economical manner in which the brain might effect pattern recognition immediately suggests experiments that could test the validity of the model. For instance, the model discussed above would imply that, up to a point, the recognition of a large pattern should be more rapid than the recognition of a similar small pattern. The model also suggests that the identification of the smaller of two concentric patterns may become difficult under certain conditions. In the model, recognition depends upon the spread of waves across a neural net. Because neurones possess refractory periods, one would expect a spreading wave of excitation to be unable to pass through a region of the network in which elements had recently been active. Thus if two concentric identical figures were exposed consecutively, the smaller one first, the smaller figure should not be perceived, since the spread of waves necessary for its identification could not pass through the refractory region left by exposure of the second and larger pattern. There is evidence that something of the sort occurs in human vision. Werner (1935) found that when he presented a small black disk and a concentric black ring consecutively in the visual field, an observer could fail to see the ring if the stimulus interval lay between 12–25 msec; in Werner's experiments, the outer border of the disk and the inner border of the ring were coincident. This phenomenon has been called 'visual masking', and has been further studied by Kolers & Rosner (1960). They exposed the disk and the ring (*D* and *R* of the inset to Fig. 52*a*) separately, one to each eye in sequence; the fact that they confirmed Werner's observations (Fig. 52*a*) suggests that visual masking has a cortical origin. They also found that the stimulus interval providing the maximal masking of the disk increased with increase of *d*,

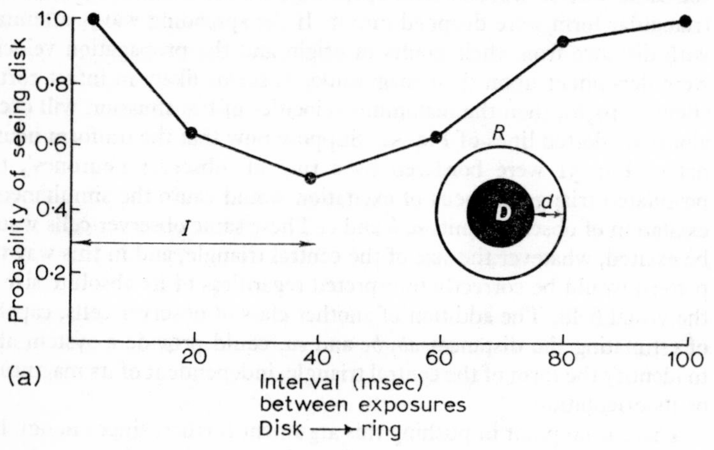

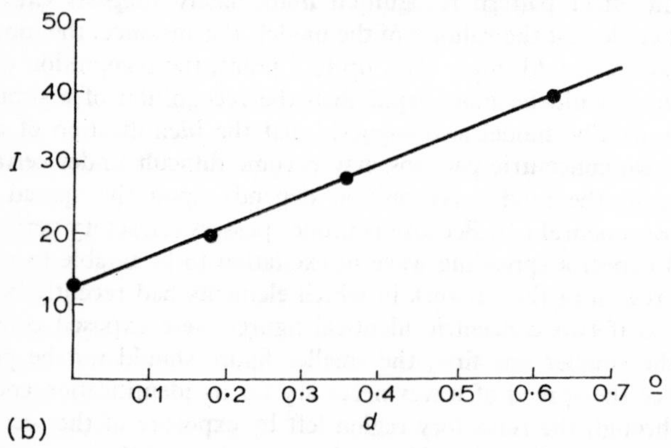

FIG. 52. The dependence of visual masking upon the angular separation, *d* of a disk, *D*, and surrounding circle, *R*.

(*a*) Disk and ring presented for 35 msec each with $d = 0{\cdot}62°$. I = estimated interval giving maximal masking (or minimal probability of seeing the disk).

(*b*) The relation between *I* and *d*. For further details, see text. (From results of Kolers & Rosner, 1960, *Am. J. Psychol.*, **73**, 2.)

the angular separation of disk from ring. By interpreting their results with a little artistic licence, one obtains the graph drawn in Fig. 52*b*, which indicates a rectilinear relationship between optimal stimulus interval for masking and *d*. Although the calculation is necessarily uncertain, it is interesting to estimate the probable cortical transmission velocity implied by Fig. 52*b*. On the wave-theory of pattern recognition these results would imply that excitation was spreading out from the focus of excitation produced by the borders of the disk at the rate of some 0·0225°/msec. Daniel & Whitteridge (1961) found that 5·6 mm cortex represented 1° of foveal visual field for the monkey. If we assume that a similar value holds for man, then Kolers and Rosner's results would imply a transcortical transmission velocity of about 0·12 m/sec. It is almost embarrassing that an estimate which involved so many assumptions and employed, without shame, data from man, monkey and cat should come so close to the observed transmission velocity of the burst response in isolated cortex (p. 63).

There is evidence that the masking referred to above, of one circular figure by another, is not restricted to patterns of this form. Averbach & Sperling (1960) reported that when the brief exposure of a letter to one eye is followed by presentation of a 'surrounding' circle to the other eye, the enclosed letter is not perceived. They were studying short-term storage of information in vision and considered this to represent ". . . a quick substitution of the circle for the stored letter". They referred to 'erasure' of the letter by the circle and were apparently unaware of Kolers and Rosner's study of visual masking.

Retinal visual codes

The various speculative arguments above should have made it clear that we are still a long way from understanding the codes in which information about the visual field is transmitted from the visual cortex for use by the rest of the brain. Even if the same central code is used by different species, it seems likely that the spatial summations necessary to an appropriate behaviour of cortical neurones may occur in different parts of the visual system for different species. No one has yet reported movement-sensitive ganglion cells in the cat's retina; on the other hand, such cells have been described in the frog (Maturana, Lettvin, McCulloch & Pitts, 1960) and in the rabbit (Barlow, Hill & Levick, 1964). Table 2 may give some idea of the presently apparent variation between species.

Some of these recorded differences may ultimately prove to be the consequence of different experimental techniques, the care with which they were used, or different interpretations of similar data. For instance, Barlow, Hill and Levick believe that the 'movement gated convexity detectors' of frogs, described by Lettvin *et al.* (1959) may be identical

TABLE 2

Functional types of optic nerve fibre that have been described

Species	*Functional types described*	*Author*	*Date*
Frog	ON; OFF; ON–OFF	Hartline	1938
Frog	Convexity and net-dimming detectors	Lettvin *et al.*	1959
Cat	Concentric ON-centre with OFF surround, and vice versa	Kuffler	1953
Pigeon	Movement and horizontal edge detectors	Maturana & Frenk	1963
Rabbit	As for cat, above, and movement detectors; also slow movement detectors	Barlow *et al.*	1964

to the movement-sensitive units of rabbits, the central response of which is very easily inhibited by illumination of the peripheral receptive field. Barlow *et al.* (1964) say, "The greater response of these units to small objects is simply the consequence of inhibition from the surround caused by large objects that extend beyond the borders of the receptive field. The response has nothing to do with 'convexity' as such: frogs are interested in flies, not the mathematical abstractions that preoccupied the investigators."

The difficulties of breaking the code by which sensory information is transmitted are the same, whether one is studying the visual system at the cortical or the retinal level. Progress is not so much retarded by the technical difficulties of making accurate measurements, as it is by our not knowing which of many possible tests to make. "The response to static spots of light turned on and off enables one to differentiate 'on-off' units from the others, but one has to test with moving spots to understand that these units signal the direction of motion of objects in the visual field. If one's apparatus is inflexible, or if one's attention is too narrowly confined to the problem of differentiating classes of units, one may easily omit the relatively crude observations and experiments that tell one most clearly what are the triggering features, and hence reveal most about the code. . . . The scissors, string and shadows on the wall required to answer the questions that arise at this stage may resemble the equipment for a children's party more than scientific apparatus, but the answers are necessary before more quantitative analysis becomes worthwhile." (Barlow, Hill & Levick, 1964.)

Transmission of information in the brain

Studies of learning in experimental animals have made it clear that virtually any part of the mammalian brain can be functionally connected to any other part. Although this has long been an established fact of experimental psychology, until recently there was little evidence from neurophysiological work to suggest that excitation could spread from any part of the brain to any other. Neurophysiological observation in this field has been hampered by the presence of spontaneous activity, the common usage of large recording electrodes and by anaesthesia. Nevertheless, Buser, Borenstein & Bruner (1959) demonstrated in cats under chloralose anaesthesia electrical responses to visual and auditory stimuli in parts of the cerebral cortex that were some distance from the primary receiving areas. In their experiments, evoked responses were recorded with surface electrodes and were averaged by superimposing photographs (p. 35).

More recently, Burns & Smith (1962) have investigated the spread of excitation within the isolated forebrain of the unanaesthetized cat. Extracellular micropipettes were used to record the activity of cortical units, and the response of single neurones to excitation of distant parts of the brain's surface was estimated from the post-stimulus histogram. In this case, the post-stimulus histogram represented the average behaviour of a neurone following about 100 stimuli. A flat, or horizontal, P.S.H. could show that the unit in question was equally likely to fire at any time following a stimulus and would imply absence of response. Any clear-cut, statistically significant deviation from a horizontal P.S.H. would indicate that stimulation had modified the unit's behaviour and was taken as an indication of response (p. 44). Measured in this way, a response to the local excitation of any close-packed group of cortical cells could be demonstrated from neurones all over the accessible cerebral cortex. The test stimuli used for these experiments were either delivered direct to the cortical surface and consisted of bursts of 10 stimuli at 100/sec, repeated once every second, or consisted of a 6° white disk, focused and flashed at 1/sec upon one retina.

These experiments made it clear that in the unanaesthetized cat's brain excitation of a group of cortical cells could modify the behaviour of cortical neurones at any point in the cerebral cortex, however remote. Nevertheless, the influence of an excited, close-packed group of neurones upon a distant unit was so weak that it could usually only be distinguished from the noise of spontaneous activity by averaging the responses to about 100 stimuli at 1/sec. This fact might at first sight suggest that these observations had little relevance to the form of excitation that must spread through the normal brain and make recognition of stimuli and appropriate muscular responses possible. It is clear that the intact brain does not have to wait for 100 identical stimuli before any decision is possible about the site and nature of stimulation. A reaction time of about $\frac{1}{4}$ sec means that even a complex set of external stimuli can be identified in less than 250 msec. On the other hand, Burns and Smith's results showed that behaviour of a large number (possibly all) of cortical neurones was modified by local cortical excitation. Thus, while the information passed on by one neurone in one second is insufficient to describe the source of excitation, the information received from several hundred neurones might well justify a specific output from the nervous system after 250 msec. One has to assume that differentiation of the effects of a stimulus from the noise of 'spontaneous' activity is only made possible by the simultaneous, weak responses of many neurones.

Such a system for the transmission of information within the nervous system would depend for its efficiency upon redundancy of behaviour. Many neurones must do the same thing at the same time. Although a system that is apparently costly in a number of components, it is one with obvious advantages. Any system that relies upon the transmission of most of the available information by a relatively small number of neurones risks failure due to the degeneration of a few essential elements. In contrast, an arrangement that permits only a small fraction of the available information to be carried by each of a large number of units is unlikely to be seriously affected by the death of a few neurones; and there is good evidence that central neurones do die in small numbers every day throughout adult life (Burns, 1958). Thus, the postulate that information is transmitted from place to place within the brain as a feeble modification of the probability of discharge for large numbers of neurones, may explain the observed resistance of normal behaviour to large-scale removal of cortex (Lashley, 1929). For the same reasons, one would expect the continual degeneration of cortical neurones that appears to accompany increasing age to have little effect upon behaviour, until a large fraction of the original inhabitants of the skull had disappeared. Perhaps these considerations offer a tenable explanation of the relatively sudden onset of senile dementia, or the long-delayed appearance of post-encephalitic Parkinsonism (DeJong & Burns, 1967).

In any case, there is independent evidence that duplication of behaviour is an important feature of cortical construction. The columns of cortical neurones with similar properties, described by Mountcastle and by Hubel and Wiesel, are examples of functional redundancy.

Many neurophysiologists seem to have conducted their research in the belief that each neurone of the cerebral cortex has a specific function to perform; an individual function that could ultimately be identified, with sufficient refinement of technique. On the other hand, all of the presently available evidence suggests that philogenetic development of the brain has sought a method for the transmission of information that would be least vulnerable to local damage. A brain that reserved one nerve cell for each job would not have this reliability. It seems more likely that each neurone can transmit a very small fraction of the information contained in many aspects of the total sensory input. So far as they go, the results of statistical analysis of the behaviour of cortical units in the primary visual area and elsewhere are consistent with this expectation.

CHAPTER 6

THE STABILITY OF CORTICAL NEURONES

CORTICAL neurones in the lightly anaesthetized animal, or in the isolated, unanaesthetized forebrain, display continual or 'spontaneous' activity. Although the precise timing of individual discharges cannot be predicted with certainty, the averate rate of discharge, expressed as mean frequency per minute, remains constant for many hours, provided that the nervous system is not exposed to circulatory changes resulting from inconstant temperature, respiration or blood pressure. This statement appears to be true of neurones in the cat's primary visual cortex (Burns, Heron & Pritchard, 1962), of units in the cat's 'association areas' (Burns & Smith, 1962) and of nerve cells in the rat's cerebral cortex (Bindman, Lippold & Redfearn, 1964).

This constant rate of discharge can, in fact, be altered or reset to new levels by various, somewhat dramatic, procedures. A period of polarization of the recorded unit can alter the mean frequency of discharge to some new level which persists without change for more than an hour after the polarizing current is switched off (Bindman, Lippold & Redfearn, 1964; Burns, 1957). Some of the other methods which can be employed to reset unit frequency are discussed in the next chapter. The fact that we wish to stress here is the comparative stability of the discharge rate of cortical neurones. In general, it appears that activity of ascending afferents to the cerebral cortex redistributes the discharges of cortical units in time, but is very unlikely to alter the total number of spikes per minute (Burns, Heron & Pritchard, 1962; Bliss, Burns & Uttley, 1968).

The inflexibility of discharge rate of cortical neurones is of interest for at least two reasons. First, it implies that this parameter of their behaviour is unlikely to be of physiological importance in the recording and transmission of information by the central nervous system. Second, it suggests that the maintenance of a steady, overall level of cortical activity might be one important goal governing some of the more complex goal-seeking operations of the central nervous system. In any case, one would like to know the mechanism by which this constancy of discharge frequency is maintained, despite the continual fluctuations of afferent excitation that must occur.

Unfortunately, there seems to be little experimental evidence bearing upon this question. It is possible that the frequency of cortical units is governed by the existence of an arrangement of neurones providing negative feed-back. If each cortical neurone were part of a neural circuit similar to the Renshaw loop of the spinal cord (Eccles, Fatt & Koketsu, 1954), the observed stability of frequency could be achieved. In fact, Granit (1955) has suggested that the function of recurrent collaterals from motoneurones in the spinal cord might be to "... stabilize output frequency to the low values adapted for driving muscular tissue". The axons leaving spinal motoneurones have collaterals which supply Renshaw interneurones. Thus, the discharge of a motoneurone can excite neighbouring Renshaw cells, the output of which is, in turn, inhibitory to motoneurones, providing in this way a degree of negative feed-back.

There is some evidence that pyramidal cells of the cerebral cortex are part of a similar feed-back loop. Phillips (1959) has shown that antidromic excitation of pyramidal tracts in the lightly anaesthetized cat initiates a period of relative inexcitability among Betz cells in the motor cortex. He found that antidromic invasion of a Betz cell soma could be prevented by tetanic stimulation of the pyramidal tracts with a current strength that was just below threshold for excitation of the recorded neurone's axon (Fig. 53). With shocks to the pyramidal tracts that were just above this axon's threshold, he found that the highest frequency of stimulation that the recorded soma could follow, decreased with increase of stimulus strength. Put another way, the greater the number of pyramidal axons that were antidromically excited, the lower was the frequency with which individual somata could be driven. Such results are consistent with the idea that pyramidal cells of the cerebral cortex form part of a local negative feed-back loop in the same way as do motoneurones of the spinal cord. Moreover, it is known that the axons of pyramidal units give rise to 4–8 collaterals (Cajal, 1955). However, this is not the only possible interpretation of Phillips' results and he says that "... it should not be concluded, without some caution, that the recurrent collaterals of the pyramidal axons are alone responsible ... however tempting this may be in view of their profusion...."

Eccles, Anderson & Løyning (1963) have been less cautious in interpreting the results of experiments with pyramidal cells of the cat's hippocampus. They claim to have demonstrated here a negative feed-back loop which is exactly analogous to the Renshaw circuit, in which "... the basket cell ... corresponds to the postulated inhibitory neurone, and there is no alternative." This unequivocal interpretation of their results has been disputed by Gloor (1963) who felt that insufficient consideration had been given to alternative explanations of their results. However, if there are neurones in the cerebral cortex that function in the manner of Renshaw cells, then one of the central

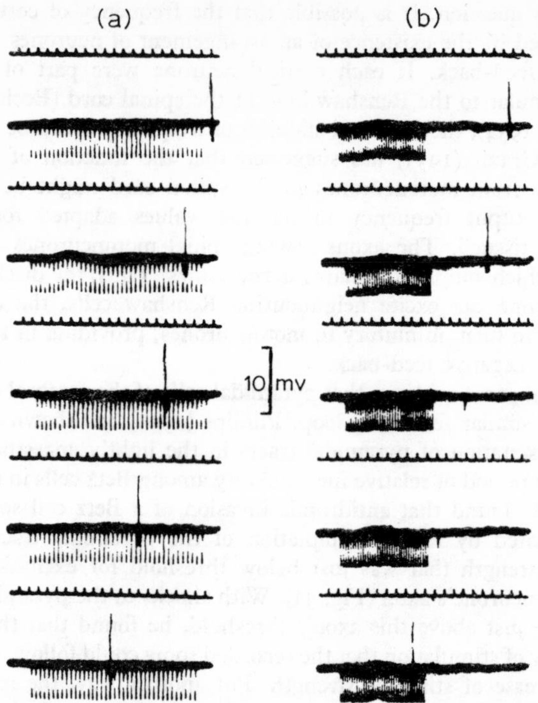

FIG. 53. Extracellular recording to show blockage of antidromic invasion by tetanic stimulation below threshold for axons of this cell.

(*a*) Antidromic tetanization with 38 shocks at 200 c/s, strength 80 μA, fails to excite the axon of this Betz cell, and does not prevent invasion of this cell by an antidromic impulse set up by a stronger (140 μA) shock. Antidromic latency, 1·35 msec.

(*b*) Antidromic tetanization with 37 shocks at 420 c/s, strength 80 μA. The testing antidromic impulse is blocked in the third and fourth records. Time, 100 c/s.

(From Phillips, 1959, *Q. Jl exp. Physiol.*, **44**, 1, Fig. 15.)

actions of atropine becomes more intelligible. The cerebral cortex of the anaesthetized cat (except with chloralose anaesthesia) liberates acetylcholine in quantities that are roughly proportional to the degree of spontaneous activity as estimated from the electrocorticogram (MacIntosh & Oborin, 1953; Mitchell, 1963). The rate of acetylcholine liberation is considerably increased by the systemic administration of atropine. If atropine were to block acetylcholine receptors upon interneurones in the postulated cortical feed-back circuit, one might expect pyramidal neurones to fire at a greater frequency since their output would no longer be capable of inhibiting their own discharge. Unfortunately, there is no evidence at present concerning the effect of systemic atropine upon the mean frequency of firing of cortical neurones.

Whatever the final outcome of this issue, present results are at least consistent with the idea that some cortical neurones are part of local feed-back circuits, and it seems possible that these circuits are responsible for the observed stability of discharge frequency. If the presence of Renshaw-type circuits within the cortex is not responsible, then some other source of negative feed-back must be found to explain this observation. In fact, any general theory concerning the cortex, regarded as a network of interconnected neurones, must take this stability of behaviour into account. For example, concepts of learning that imply positive feed-back cannot be wholly satisfactory without modification (Milner, 1957). Thus, the assumption that learning depends upon synaptic junctions that become facilitated by repeated usage, postulates a positive feed-back that would require the addition of neural circuits with different properties if the constituent neurones are to maintain a constant frequency of discharge.

The discussion above is concerned with the implications of only one parameter of the behaviour of cortical neurones—their overall steady rate of firing. We have considered this aspect of cortical function in terms of possible goal-seeking mechanisms. It seems reasonable to ask whether there are other goals, or forms of cortical stability, that are continuously being sought by the central nervous system. An answer to this question might prove helpful in understanding the physiology of learning, in that the trained animal completing a learned reaction can usefully be described as a goal-seeking instrument (Chapter 1). If we could define the stable states of the cerebral cortex, we might become clearer about those mechanisms by which a conditioned stimulus can set up a state of instability within the central nervous system. This consideration formed part of our excuse for undertaking an investigation of binocular vision, for one can regard the eye movements that lead to binocular fusion as one part of a goal-seeking operation by the visual system. The goal in this case would appear to be some particular state of neurones in the visual cortex; it seemed possible that this goal, whatever its nature, might bear some close relation to the goal sought, perhaps in other parts of the cerebral cortex, by an animal completing a learned reaction.

Our problem then (Burns & Pritchard, 1968) was to determine the nature of the goal sought by the nervous system, when aligning the eyes for proper binocular fusion. There is ample evidence that in the cat and other species both retinae project upon the visual cortex of one hemisphere (O'Leary & Bishop, 1938; Burns, Heron & Grafstein, 1960; Hubel & Wiesel, 1962). Thus, a pattern of light upon either retina can set up a corresponding spatial pattern of excitation in one visual cortex, which despite geometrical distortion (Daniel & Whitteridge, 1961) provides a point-to-point representation of the visual field. Hubel & Wiesel (1962) observed that when a cortical unit could be driven by both eyes, its receptive fields in the two eyes ". . . were similarly organized, had the same axis orientation and occupied corresponding regions in the two retinas". One would therefore imagine that identical patterns of light, projected separately upon the two retinae, would set up very similar distributions of response across the visual cortex of one hemisphere. If two such identical patterns were exposed simultaneously upon the two retinae, then the two corresponding patterns of cortical excitation would presumably overlap and interfere. With the two eyes properly aligned for binocular fusion, the resultant pattern of cortical response must have some properties that represent a goal for the visual system—a condition of stability, requiring no further change in the action of extrinsic ocular muscles. Our purpose, therefore, was to determine which aspects of the compound pattern of cortical excitation, produced by similar light–dark edges falling upon corresponding points of the two retinae, could possibly serve as the goal that determines binocular alignment for fusion in the intact animal.

This problem may be made clearer by reference to the model illustrated in Fig. 54. In this analogue of the visual system, two real images of a distant object are cast upon a screen; the light responsible for each image is reflected from a mirror and passes through a convex lens. In the model, rotation of the mirrors would represent rotations of the eyes in one plane, the lenses represent the optical systems of the eyes, while the distribution of light across the image screen provides an analogue for the distribution of excitation across one visual cortex. Such a model would be relatively realistic if it were known that the excitation fed to a cortical district from the two eyes were additive and there is evidence from the experiments described below that this is the case. In the model system it is assumed that the two mirrors are aligned for fused binocular vision, when their mutual directions are such that there is perfect overlap of the two images upon the screen. The system would continuously hunt binocular fusion, as defined above, if one of the following conditions provided a goal for the movements of its mirrors:

1. the least number of light–dark boundaries on the screen;
2. the greatest gradients of light intensity across the screen.

By analogy, one might expect the visual system in the binocular animal to be continually hunting an alignment of the eyes providing either:

1. the least number of responding cells in the visual cortex (cells firing above or below their resting level of discharge); or
2. the largest possible local responses.

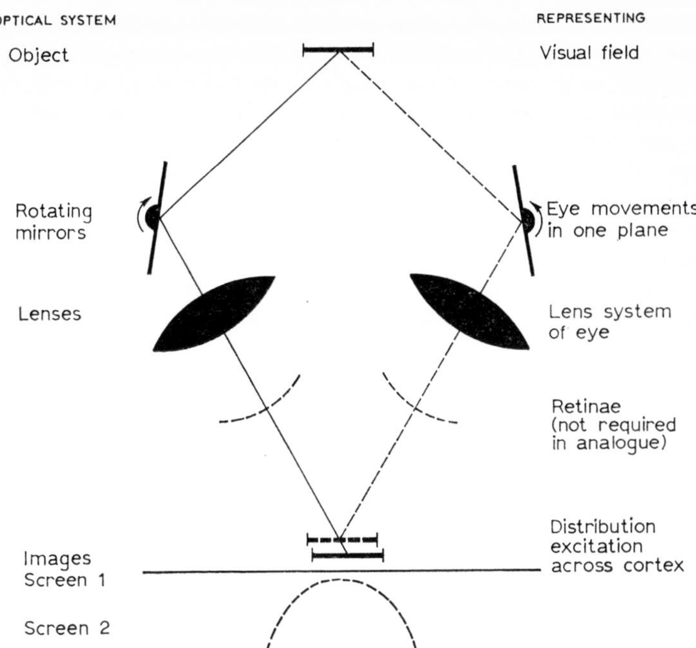

FIG. 54. Illustrating an optical analogue of a visual system providing fused binocular vision. For explanation, see text.
(From Burns & Pritchard, 1968, in preparation.)

Successful use of the second criterion would require that some units in the visual cortex exhibit spatial summation when excited by similar light–dark boundaries presented simultaneously to the two retinae. Moreover, whatever the form of this spatial summation, it should have a critical value (maximal or minimal) for a unique relative position of the exciting patterns. Successful use of the first criterion would not necessitate the presence of spatial summation.

With these considerations in mind, we tried to determine in the experimental animal the behaviour of cortical units when stimulated by similar patterns projected upon roughly corresponding parts of the two retinae. The experimental procedure was as follows.

One visual cortex was exposed in the isolated, unanaesthetized forebrain in the cat. The animal's eyes were then covered with contact glasses and fitted with 10D spectacle lenses, bringing two ground-glass screens some 30 cm in front of the animal into focus upon the two retinae. The screens provided independent fields for the two eyes; no light could reach either eye from the contralateral screen. Stimuli consisted of two straight light–dark borders, one projected upon each screen; both borders were given in-phase artificial saccadic movements consisting of rectangular oscillations at about 3 c/s with amplitude 0·5°.

Directly an apparently reliable cortical unit had been found with the micropipette, its representative district was determined separately in the ipsi- and contralateral fields. We found, as did Hubel & Wiesel (1962), that the preferred orientation of border was approximately the same for both fields. One light–dark border was placed so that it crossed the representative district of one field and thus provided maximal or near-maximal responses in the post-stimulus histogram. This border, which I shall refer to as the 'constant border', was left to oscillate in this position throughout the remainder of the experiment. A border with

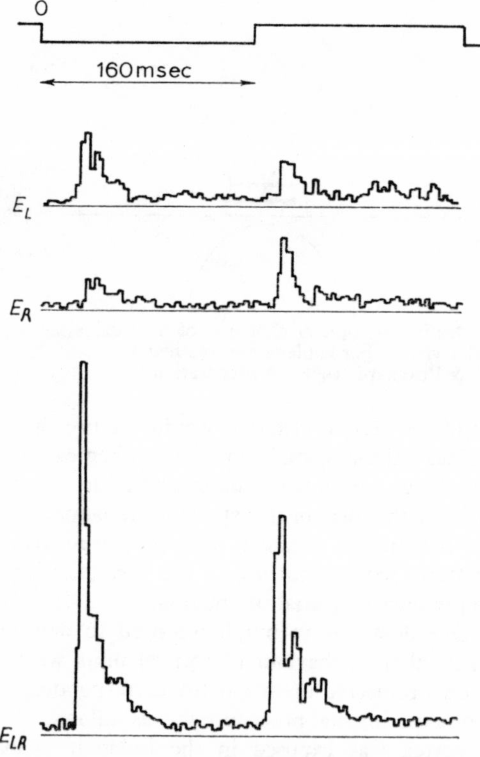

FIG. 55. The spatial summation shown by a neurone in the cat's visual cortex when excited by both eyes. The uppermost record shows the movements of straight light–dark edges in the two visual fields. E_L = average response to excitation of the left retina alone. E_R = average response to excitation of the right retina alone. E_{LR} = average response to excitation of both retinae simultaneously. Ordinates: proportional to counts per δt. Abscissae: time, as indicated by record of pattern movement. (From Burns & Pritchard, 1968, in preparation.)

the same orientation was now presented, oscillating at a variety of positions in the other field, and records were made of unit response to this form of binocular excitation. We found considerable spatial summation occurred when both borders lay near to their respective representative districts. Figure 55 shows the impressive summation that always occurs under these conditions. The upper trace shows the in-phase movements of the exciting patterns. The next two traces, marked E_L and E_R, show the responses of the cortical unit to excitation through the left and right eyes separately. The lowest record shows the response of the unit when excited by both eyes simultaneously. A more dramatic version of the same phenomenon is illustrated in Fig. 56. This unit

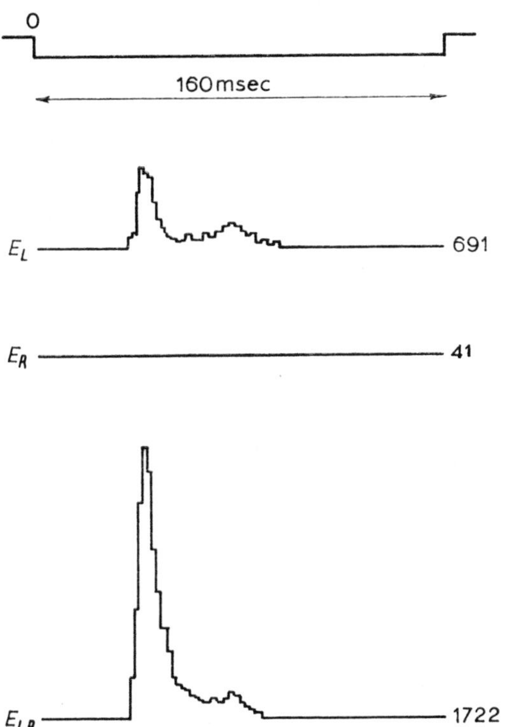

FIG. 56. A more dramatic version of the spatial summation illustrated in Fig. 55. (Records as in Fig. 55.) The numbers at the end of the histograms indicate mean discharge rates.
(From Burns & Pritchard, 1968, in preparation.)

would not respond to any form of excitation through the right eye; nevertheless, a comparison between records E_L and E_{LR} shows clearly that stimulation of the right eye raised the excitability of the cell. Units with these properties are relatively easy to find, but we have also encountered cells whose behaviour could apparently only be influenced by one retina. Hubel & Wiesel (1962) reported evidence of binocular convergence for only 84% of cells tested. One might expect this figure to be increased in experiments without anaesthesia and in which statistical measures of response were employed, but we have no reliable estimates to offer. We simply concluded from these experiments that the majority of neurones in the visual cortex receives excitatory connections from both retinae, and exhibits spatial summation of excitation whenever light–dark borders with the same orientation cross corresponding parts of the two visual fields.

The preceding experimental results satisfy one demand of the second criterion discussed on p. 123, namely that spatial summation of the excitations received from the two retinae occurs in the visual cortex.

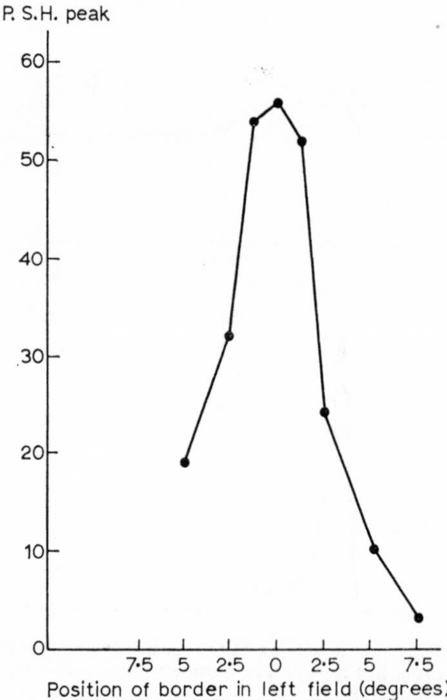

FIG. 57. Variation of unit response with position of a straight, black–white border in the field viewed by the left eye. The right eye was always observing a similar constant border, oscillating across the representative district. The orientations of both borders were the same and both moved in phase.
(From Burns & Pritchard, 1968, in preparation.)

Successful use by the nervous system of this criterion also required that any form of spatial summation employed as a goal by the visual system should have a unique critical value. Figure 57 shows that this is so. The results for this curve were obtained while a constant border was exhibited in the right field, passing through the representative district with the same orientation as the test border used to explore the left field. Thus, while the constant border was always in the same place, the border projected upon the left screen was presented in a variety of positions as for the monocular tests. The results show that there is only one relative position for the left and right borders which excites a maximal response; this occurs when both borders pass through their representative districts.

It is convenient to describe similar patterns with this *relative* position in the two visual fields as 'aligned', whether or not the borders actually pass through the representative districts. Thus, if two borders are first arranged to pass through the left and right representative districts and then both are moved by the same angular displacement, in the same direction, they would still be described as aligned. The use of this terminology assumes that if the borders are aligned so that they both pass through the representative districts of one cortical unit, they will pass through the left and right representative districts for all similar neurones in the visual cortex. Figure 58 shows that peak cortical excitation is greater for patterns that are properly aligned than it is for the same patterns when misaligned. We have already pointed out (p. 92) how curves like those of Fig. 58 provide a measure of the distribution of excitation across the cerebral cortex, produced in a network of similar cells by a pattern exposed in one part of the visual field. If this interpretation of such curves is accepted, then Fig. 58 indicates the distributions of excitation across the cortex produced by aligned and misaligned patterns. Aligned patterns appear to evoke a greater local response over a considerable area surrounding the peak of excitation, than do misaligned patterns.

It seems likely that successful fusion of binocular vision in the cat requires equivalent borders in the two visual fields to be aligned, at least for a majority of cortical neurones representing central vision. But there is no proof of this; nor can there be from the sort of experiment described above. All that these experiments show is that, given a simple pattern in the visual field, there is a unique alignment of the eyes producing a maximal response from cortical units. If this unique relative position of the two eyes is that adopted during fusion in the intact animal, then either maximum peak local response or maximal tangential gradient of excited cortex might serve as goals for eye movements seeking binocular fusion.

In any case, it would be quite impossible to determine whether either

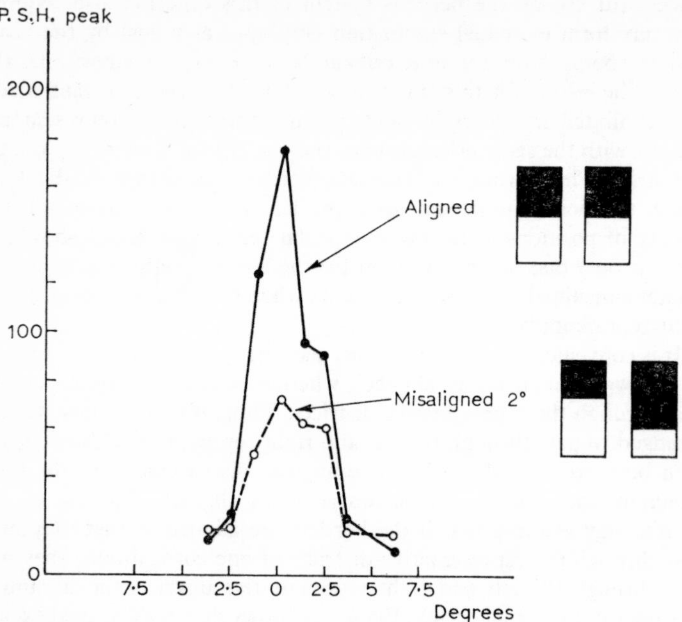

FIG. 58. Variation of unit response with position of two similar borders exposed in the fields of left and right eyes. The orientations of the borders were the same, and both moved in phase.
(From Burns & Pritchard, 1968, in preparation.)

of these factors did serve as a criterion for satisfactory fusion from experiments of the sort described above. In such animal preparations all eye movements are prevented with gallamine; moreover, the surgery for isolating the forebrain severs neural connections that are essential to this goal-seeking operation. However, such hypotheses derived from experiments with acute preparations occasionally provide unexpected predictions about behaviour in the intact animal that can be readily tested. One observation from our work with the cat's isolated forebrain proved extremely useful in this respect. We found that aligned, straight light–dark edges produced a minimal response from cortical units when these patterns were presented to the two eyes with relative orientations of 180° (Fig. 59). (This means, for example, if the left were excited by a pattern that was light above and dark below, the right retina would be exposed to a parallel border, separating dark above from light below.) Only when the patterns were slightly misaligned in either direction did binocular excitation produce a clear two-peaked response (Fig. 60).

The implication of this finding is that the intact animal, presented

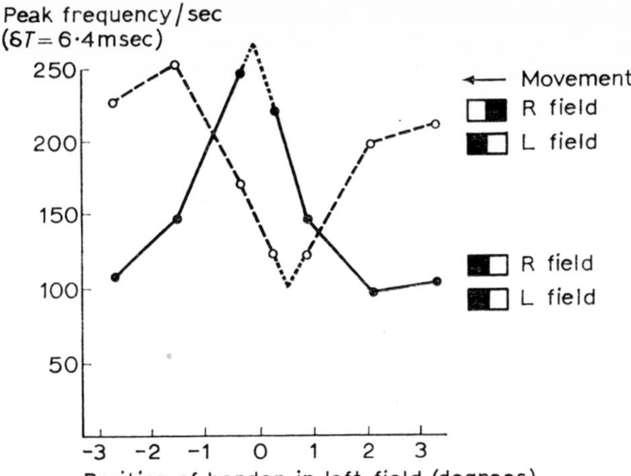

FIG. 59. The variation of unit response with position of a pair of aligned, light–dark edges, presented simultaneously to the left and right eyes. ●——● shows response when the patterns were similar. O - - - O shows response when the patterns were mutually inverted.
(From Burns & Pritchard, 1968, in preparation.)

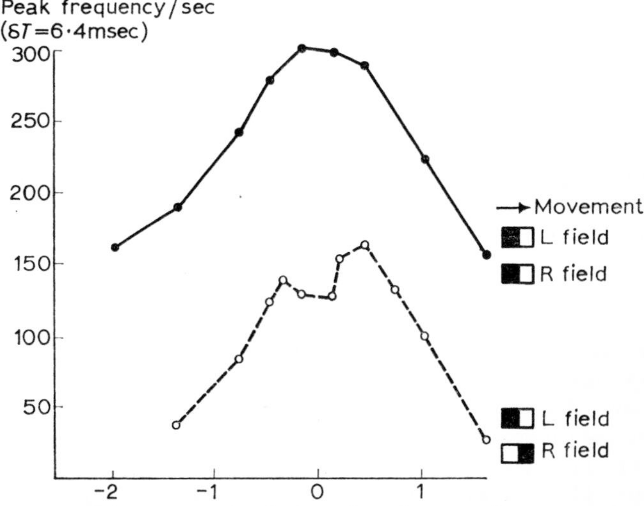

FIG. 60. The variation of unit response with position of a pair of parallel, light–dark edges, presented simultaneously to the left and right eyes. ●——● shows response when the patterns were similar. O - - - O shows response when the patterns were mutually inverted. In both cases the patterns were misaligned by about 0·5°.
(From Burns & Pritchard, 1968, in preparation.)

with the same inverted patterns, should misalign its eyes if alignment for normal fusion requires some aspect of the cortical response to be maximal. It would be extremely difficult to test this prediction in the cat, but comparatively easy to do so in man. Consequently we turned our attention to human subjects and proceeded on the assumption that processes governing binocular fusion were likely to be the same in both species. The method employed was as follows.

Subjects were seated comfortably at a table, using a bite-bar to steady the position and orientation of the head. They viewed two ground-glass screens through a mirror stereoscope arranged so that neither eye could see the contralateral field. Straight, horizontal light–dark borders were projected upon the two screens in such a way that one visual field was dark above and light below, while the pattern on the other was inverted, with light above and dark below. One border was left in the same position, about mid-screen, for the whole experiment; the other border was presented to the subject in a variety of positions. When the two borders were at different altitudes, the observer invariably reported a three-part field—either a black band upon a grey background or a white band upon a darker background—depending on the polarity of this difference in altitude. When the borders were nearly, or exactly, in line, all observers reported one of two percepts. Either:

a. there was a dominance of one eye and only one field was perceived, or

b. a three-part field was reported, consisting of a thin black or white line upon a grey background.

Since, for the purpose of this study, we were not interested in conditions leading to ocular dominance, we disregarded reports that only one field has been seen. (Unfortunately, the relative frequencies of percepts *a* and *b* were not recorded; it is probable, however, that *a* was somewhat more common than *b*.)

No subject was informed of the relative altitudes of the two borders, a variety of which was presented in random order. Directly the position of the edges was arranged, the subjects were asked to open their eyes and estimate the width and relative brightness of the central bar (if they saw a three-part field) from a millimetre scale which was presented in one field only. The results of such an experiment are shown in Fig. 61. The abscissa shows the actual relative displacement of the borders. The ordinate shows the subject's estimate of width for the central bar; the upper half of the diagram implies reports of a white bar upon a grey background, while entries in the lower half indicate that a black bar upon a light background was seen. For comparison, each subject was tested in the same way with light–dark borders of the same orientation (both fields contained, say, black above and white

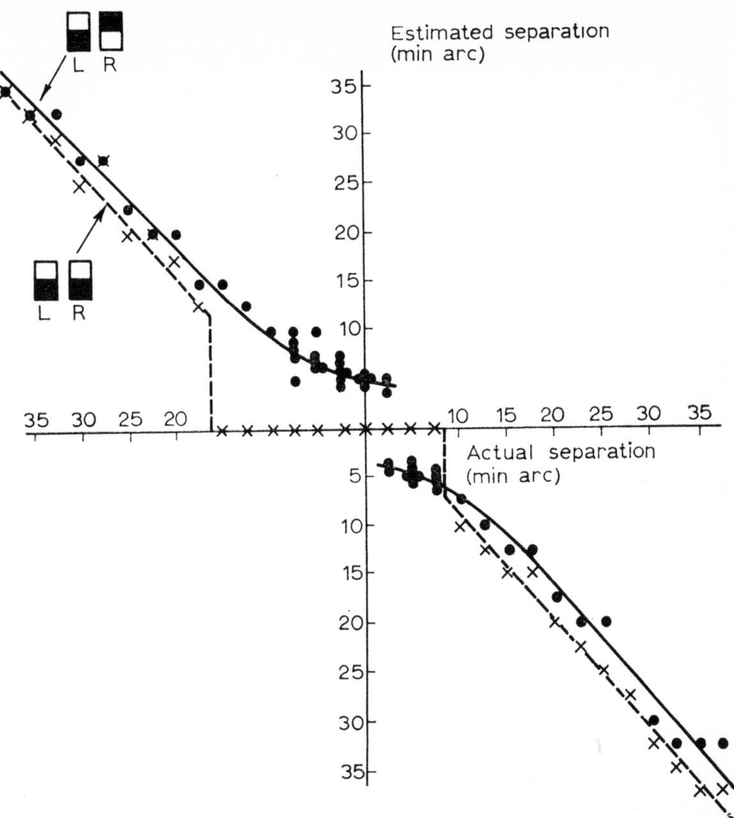

FIG. 61. The relation between actual separation and the separation estimated by a human observer of two parallel, horizontal light–dark borders, viewed simultaneously in the fields of left and right eyes. X - - - X shows the results for similar orientations. ●——● shows results obtained when the patterns were mutually inverted.
(From Burns & Pritchard, 1968, in preparation.)

below) and all showed the expected fusion of borders that were presented within some 30 min arc of one another (Ogle, 1950).

The results obtained with inverted patterns were consistent with the prediction made from experiments on the cat's isolated forebrain. They could be interpreted as demonstrating that when inverted patterns are presented with the borders nearly or exactly in line, the visual system seeks a misalignment of the eyes in order to produce some aspect of maximal excitation in the visual cortex. That the subject's eyes were in fact misaligned under these conditions was demonstrated in the following way. The horizontal borders of the two inverted patterns were first placed at the same altitude and consequently lay along a single straight line. A fine wire was now stretched horizontally across the two ground-glass screens, on the side away from the observer. This wire could be illuminated by a 0·02 sec flash of light so that its shadow fell exactly along both borders. When a subject observing the inverted black–white borders as before, reported a three-part field, the wire shadow was flashed upon the screens. All subjects viewing under these conditions reported that they had perceived two wire shadows, separated by approximately the width of the thin centre bar in their three-part field. The same subjects, when presented with identical left and right patterns of the same orientation, invariably reported a single wire shadow whenever they had achieved fusion of the two fields.

These experiments imply that both the cat and the human, when seeking binocular fusion, are hunting for a relative direction of the eyes that will provide a maximal value for some aspect of excitation in the visual cortex. The results of the human experiment described above make it quite clear that the goal sought cannot be a minimum number of light–dark borders in the fused percept—implying a minimum number of separate peaks of excitation in the visual cortex. It seems that the nervous system must seek either peak local excitation or maximal gradient of excitation across the network of neurones in the visual cortex, or some other parameter of maximal local response. Consequently, we tried to design an experiment on human subjects that might assess the relative importance to binocular fusion of peak excitation and spread of excitation in the visual cortex.

The results of these experiments, which are described below, indicated that peak local excitation was not the goal sought, and that the nervous system is probably hunting a maximal gradient of cortical excitation in its attempts to achieve fusion. This interpretation assumes, of course, that responses to retinal excitation are similar in the visual cortex of cat and man.

Subjects were presented as before with independent left and right fields, viewed through a mirror stereoscope. A black rectangular bar upon a grey background was presented in the right field; the left visual field contained a parallel, white bar of the same dimensions seen against a black background. Illumination of the two fields was the same. Subjects were presented with the two targets at a variety of angular separations and asked to estimate the apparent separation of the right-hand edges of these targets in the binocular field, in the manner described for the experiment of Fig. 61. Figure 62 shows the results obtained, plotted in the same way as for Fig. 61.

This experiment suggests that maximal gradient of cortical excitation is the goal sought during binocular fixation. Figure 63 illustrates our

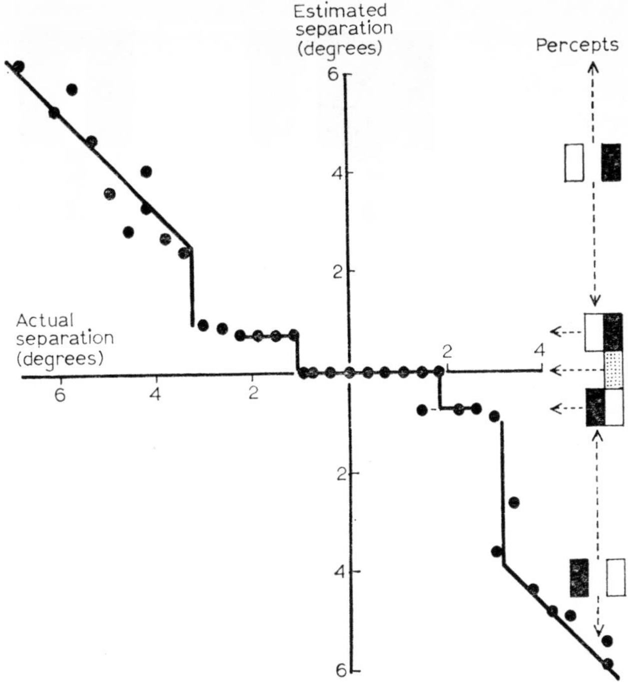

FIG. 62. The relation between actual separation and the separation estimated by a human observer of two vertical bars, viewed simultaneously in the fields of left and right eyes. The left eye viewed a white bar upon a black background. The right eye viewed a black bar upon a grey background. The bars were 42 min arc wide.
(From Burns & Pritchard, 1968, in preparation.)

interpretation of these results. Figure 63*a* indicates the alignment of the two eyes, while Fig. 63*b* shows the sum of the corresponding contributions from the two fields to light intensity in the binocular field. It is assumed that the cortex is only excited by light–dark boundaries on the retinae and that this excitation is in proportion to the intensity gradients across these boundaries. For simplicity, it is assumed that the distribution of cortical response around each focus of excitation is 'triangular' and attenuates rectilinearly with increase of distance from the central peak. The contributions to cortical excitation from each edge in the binocular field are indicated by the interrupted lines of Fig. 63*c*. The continuous lines of Fig. 63*c* show an estimate of the net distribution of excitation across the visual cortex, assuming spatial summation to be algebraic for misaligned edges, but 2 × algebraic for aligned edges. This convention represents an attempt to parallel our

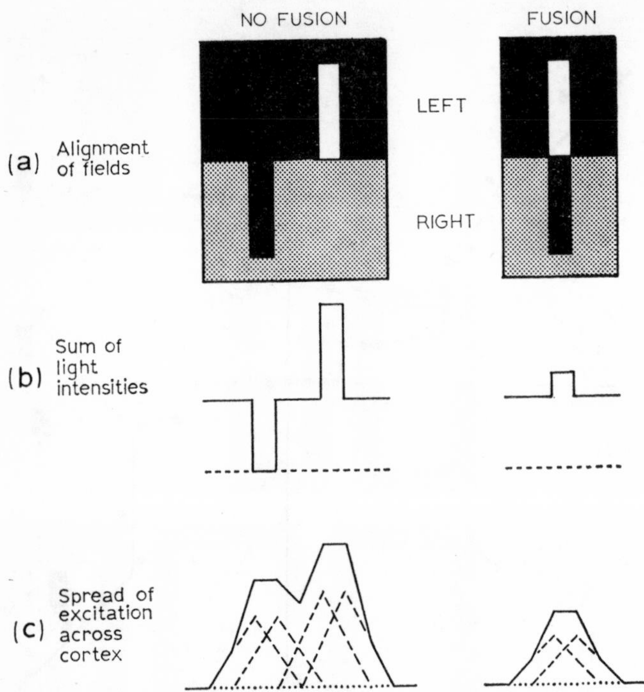

FIG. 63. An explanation of the physiological mechanism underlying the results of Fig. 62. It is supposed that binocular fusion is achieved when alignment of the eyes produces the greatest local excitation of cerebral cortex, restricted to the minimum cortical area.

observations in the cat, but is not essential to the argument. Interpreted in this way, it becomes clear that the fusion mechanism must seek maximal cortical excitation confined to the least possible cortical area; peak cortical excitation would not be the goal sought. Put in another way, the nervous system prefers a faint single percept to the percept of two bars of high contrast.

A rather similar experiment with different targets provided results that could be interpreted in the same way. In this test, the left field contained two adjacent, parallel-sided, vertical strips of illumination—one grey, one white—seen against a black background. The right field contained an identical target, so arranged that the half-targets nearest to one another were of the same intensity; either both nasal halves were white (Fig. 64*a*), or both were grey (Fig. 64*b*). One target remained in the same place throughout an experiment, while the other was exposed at a number of different positions in the same horizontal plane. Subjects were asked to describe the nature of the fused percept and to

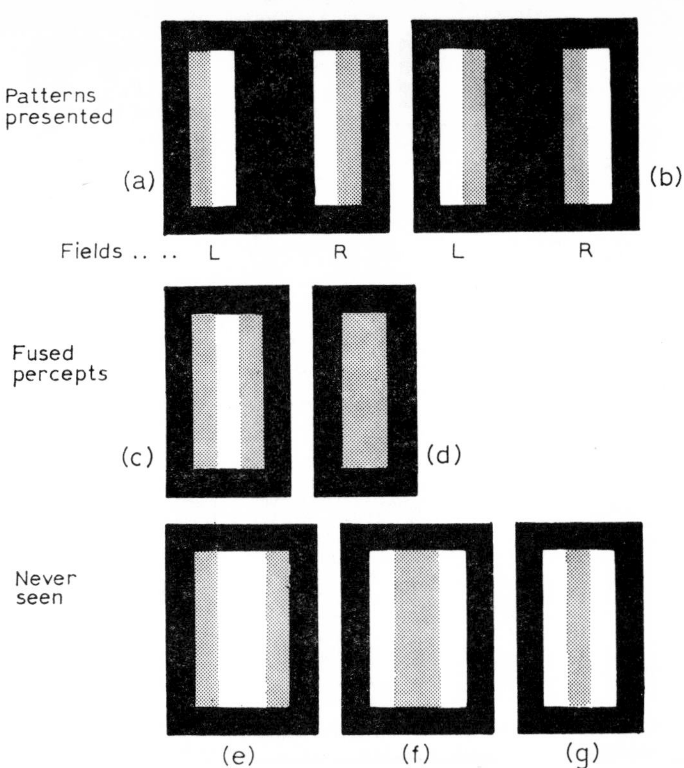

FIG. 64

(*a*) and (*b*) The grey–white patterns presented to human subjects for viewing through a mirror stereoscope.
(*c*) and (*d*) Illustrate the fused percepts that were reported.
(*e*) to (*g*) Illustrate percepts that were never reported.

estimate the apparent distances between the centres of the two grey–white strips from a scale visible in one field. Thus, when the angular separation of the targets (measured from the observer) was great, he would perceive two separate targets and the observed pattern would be reported as 'targets separate' with a sequence from left to right of either 'grey–white–black–white–grey' (GWBWG) or 'white–grey–black–grey–white' (WGBGW). The results obtained from five observers were essentially the same. The results for an observer, tested with white on the nasal side of both fields, are shown in Fig. 65. Results were similar when the grey halves of both targets were nasal. As in Fig. 61, the abscissa indicates the actual separation of the targets; the ordinate shows the subject's estimate of the separation of the mid lines of the targets. Provided that the targets were so far apart that no binocular

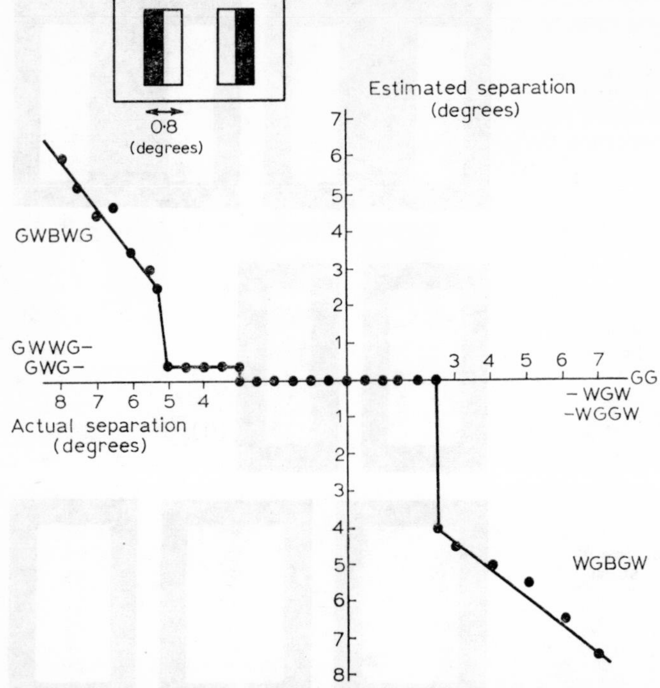

FIG. 65. The relation between actual separation and the separation estimated by a human observer of two vertical grey–white bars, viewed simultaneously in the fields of left and right eyes. Both grey–white bars were 0·8° wide. The percepts associated with various ordinate levels are indicated in capital letters.

(From Burns & Pritchard, 1967, unpublished data.)

fusion occurred, the subjects gave estimates of separation that corresponded closely with the actual separation. Fusion is indicated by the horizontal sections of the graph in Fig. 65. Only two forms of fusion were ever reported; these were either:

a. one three-strip target appearing from left to right as grey–white–grey (GWG), all the strips being of equal width (Fig. 64*c*); or

b. one two-strip target appearing as grey–grey (GG), with or without a faint black or white, very thin line down the middle (Fig. 64*d*).

The fused percepts always appeared as an integral number of strip widths. No subject ever reported any of the following:

1. a single four-strip target appearing as either grey–white–white–grey, or as white–grey–grey–white (Fig. 64*e* and *f*);
2. a single three-strip target appearing as white–grey–white (Fig. 64*g*).

The results of this experiment can be interpreted in much the same way as those of the preceding experiment. Figure 66*c* shows an estimate of the distribution of net cortical activity, produced by the binocular field when the eyes are aligned close to a GWG fusion and when their alignment produces perfect fusion. The method of calculating the hypothetical curves of Fig. 66*c* is the same as that employed in deriving

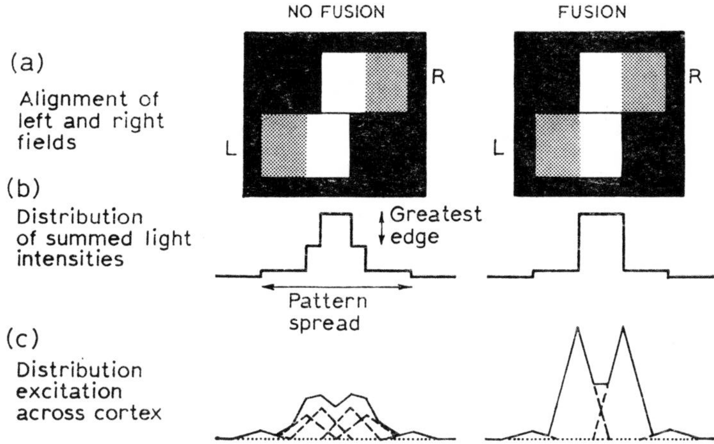

FIG. 66. An explanation of the physiological mechanism underlying the results of Figs. 64 and 65. It is supposed that binocular fusion is achieved when alignment of the eyes produces the greatest local excitation of cerebral cortex, restricted to the minimum cortical area.

Fig. 63*c*. The figure is intended to illustrate the way in which the 'cortical image' is sharpened by rotation of the eyes from near fusion to perfect GWG fusion.

It would be convenient to this argument if one could make a realistic estimate of the distribution of cortical excitation appropriate to the various percepts of this experiment. Unfortunately, this cannot be done; one would require accurate knowledge of the distributions portrayed as triangles (interrupted lines) in Fig. 66*c*; moreover, the rules of spatial summation would have to be available. Nevertheless, a crude guide to the true gradients of cortical excitation can be obtained by measuring for each relative position of the eyes:

$$\frac{\text{Greatest edge}}{\text{Pattern spread}}$$

as indicated in Fig. 66*b*. This estimate of cortical excitation gradient is plotted against relative eye position in Fig. 67. The relative eye positions providing the various percepts illustrated in Fig. 64 are indicated along

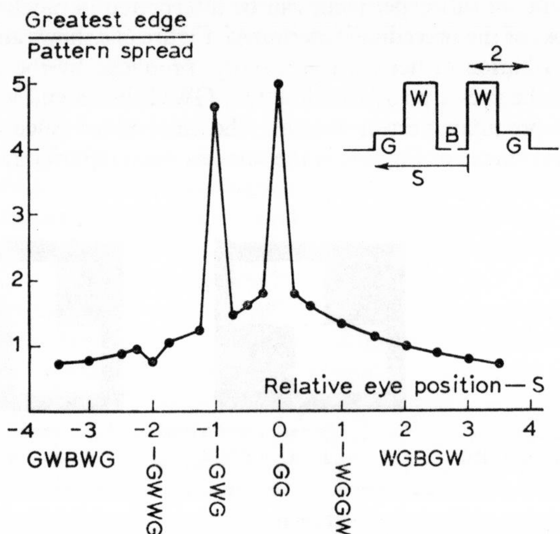

FIG. 67. A theoretical prediction of those relative eye positions that should give stable binocular fusion of the grey–white patterns of Fig. 64 (*a*) or (*b*). For further explanation, see text.
(From Burns & Pritchard, 1967, unpublished data.)

the abscissa. The two maximae opposite GWG and GG offer a ready explanation of the observed stability of these two percepts, assuming that the visual system is continuously hunting a maximal cortical excitation gradient. Moreover, the same reasoning would explain the observed absence of the percepts GWWG, WGW and WGGW, since eye positions providing these would necessarily be unstable. One would expect the GWWG percept to be the least stable of these last three. It is interesting that one out of six subjects tested, who had remarkable voluntary control over his relative eye positions and found it unusually easy to fuse stereoscopic drawings without the aid of a stereoscope, could 'force' himself to see WGGW, but could never manage to do the same for GWWG.

The hypothesis that the visual system is continually seeking a maximal gradient of cortical excitation also gains some support from the well-known suppression of response to one visual field when there is a conflict between the two fields. Suppression, or the dominance of one eye, has already been referred to in connection with the experiments of Fig. 61 in which inverted, straight black–white borders were employed as targets. A subject faced with two such fields, when the two black–white borders are in a straight line (so that one field is the negative image of the other), either misaligns his eyes or suppresses vision through one eye. If the act of suppression were to prevent in some way the arrival at the visual cortex of the input from one retina, the nervous system would have achieved the goal of maximal cortical excitation gradient, just as this goal appears to be attained by the alternative solution of ocular misalignment. Unfortunately, at present nothing is known of the site or neurophysiological nature of suppression.

Whatever the true nature of suppression, these laboratory experiments have implications for ophthalmological practice. It has been said about the treatment of diplopia (Costenbader, 1958) that ". . . suppression is the greatest single barrier to attaining secure binocular single vision". The recommended treatment consists in either blurring vision by the dominant eye (with cellophane tape or nail varnish on one spectacle lens), or increasing the illumination of the suppressed field when using binocular instruments for treatment. Our evidence suggests that the latter treatment should be effective, but the former would be very unlikely to cause significant improvement in binocular fusion. It would seem that the proper treatment should be to provide the patient with spectacles that reduce, without blurring, the light entering the dominant eye.

One other consideration makes more credible the hypothesis that the visual system is continually hunting conditions providing a maximal gradient of excitation across the visual cortex. The visual system possesses two other well-known and simple reflex responses: the fixation reflex and accommodation of the lens. The same goal that we have suggested controls the eye movements needed for fusion, would serve as an adequate end-point for these two reflexes. (Incidentally, neither of the other two goals that were considered earlier—a minimum number of peaks of maximal excitation in the visual cortex, or maximal cortical excitation itself—could operate as satisfactory goals for all three reflexes.) In the optical analogue of Fig. 54, behaviour simulating the fixation reflex could be obtained by using a curved image-screen, convex toward the lenses (screen 2 of Fig. 54). The images of off-centre objects would then be out of focus and would parallel the cortical 'defocus' of the visual system which must result from the sharing of visual afferents by light-sensitive cells in the periphery of the retina. This anatomical arrangement would necessarily increase the cortical excitation gradient as light–dark borders shift toward the retinal fovea. Thus, provided that the power of the lenses and the rotation of the mirrors in the optical analogue of Fig. 54 were controlled by a search for maximum intensity gradients upon the curved image-screen 2, this optical model would display all three simple reflexes shown by the mammalian visual system.

The reader may wonder why I have devoted so many pages to the description of subjective experiments in a monograph mainly concerned with the physiology of individual central neurones. The reason is that this series of observations enables one to build a precarious bridge between the properties of single units and behaviour of the whole nervous system in the intact animal. Moreover, the experimental results described in this and the preceding chapter make possible some important generalizations about cortical function. They have indicated two aspects of cortical excitation which could be regarded as goals sought by the nervous system as a whole. These are constant mean frequency of discharge for all cortical units and maximal tangential gradients of excitation within the cortical network. These two criteria of stability are probably not unconnected. The mean frequency of any individual cortical unit must be very dependent upon the behaviour of all other cortical cells. We have already seen in Chapter 5 that the presence of a light–dark border in one visual field excites some units in the visual cortex, while it inhibits their neighbours. If this is the code of behaviour by which these central neurones indicate the position of edges in the visual field, it is a code which is admirably suited to the maintenance of constant mean frequency in other parts of the brain. One would also imagine that the discharge frequency of nerve cells outside the visual cortex will be less influenced by the excitation of a remote, restricted region of visual cortex than it will be by widespread evoked responses. Our evidence suggests that binocular fusion is achieved when the excited area of visual cortex is minimal, or the cortical excitation gradients are greatest. However, there is no evidence at present to suggest that a need for maximal gradients of cortical excitation influences the behaviour of other sensory systems—although one's dislike of a discord produced by the playing of two notes separated by a semi-tone might have a similar origin!

There must certainly be many other goals sought by the nervous system and other parameters of cortical behaviour which can be legitimately regarded as stable states. A search for these stable states should prove most rewarding for, once they can be defined, we should be in a much better position to describe and understand behaviour of the intact animal.

CHAPTER 7

LEARNING AND MEMORY

Theory of learning machines

One of the most common assumptions is that learning depends upon the presence of central synapses which display a long-lasting facilitation, or increase in conductivity, directly dependent upon repeated previous usage (Eccles, 1953, 1964; Hebb, 1949). Even when not directly stated, the same hypothesis seems to be implied in the writings of those who have studied the relatively short-lasting post-tetanic potentiations that occur in the peripheral (Brown & Euler, 1938; Larrabee & Bronk, 1938) or central nervous systems (Adrian, 1936; Eccles & McIntyre, 1953). The fact that the potentiations described in these works are too transient to account for learning certainly does not rule them out as models, for similar phenomena operating upon an extended time scale may well prove responsible for the more enduring changes in behaviour of the intact animal.

A more serious objection (Burns, 1958; Young, 1964) is that learning of the form represented by conditioned reflexes requires heterosynaptic facilitation. It presupposes that activity in one pathway, X_1Y of Fig. 68,

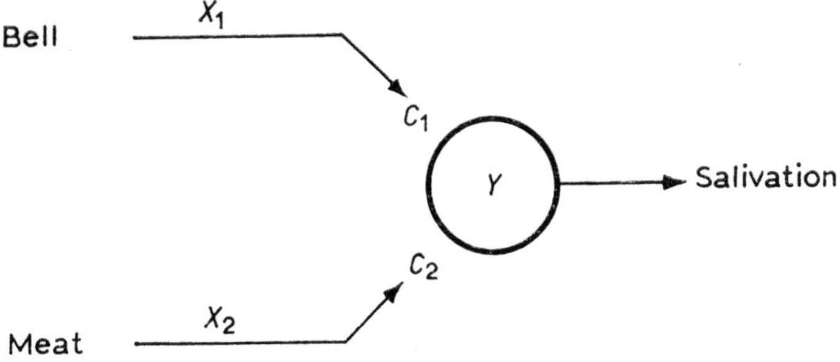

FIG. 68. The classes of neural pathway involved in formation of a conditioned reflex.

must produce after-effects in a separate, parallel pathway X_2Y. In fact, it is usually stated that repeated excitation of the class of pathway represented by X_1Y, followed by excitation of X_2Y, ultimately leads to an increase of C_1, the conductivity of the junction between X_1 and Y—

that is to say, an increase in the probability that a signal in X_1 will 'cause' a signal in Y. Thus, any changes in C_1 that occur during learning cannot be the result of activity in the $(X_1—Y)$ pathway alone. They must be caused by the past history of the *relative* activities of X_1, X_2 and Y. This necessary dependence of synaptic conductivities upon the relative activity of neurones was first clearly stated by Uttley (1956).

He (Uttley, 1954) had already described the logical requirements of a machine designed for the classification of input signals. An example of his classification system is provided in Fig. 69. It is supposed that both

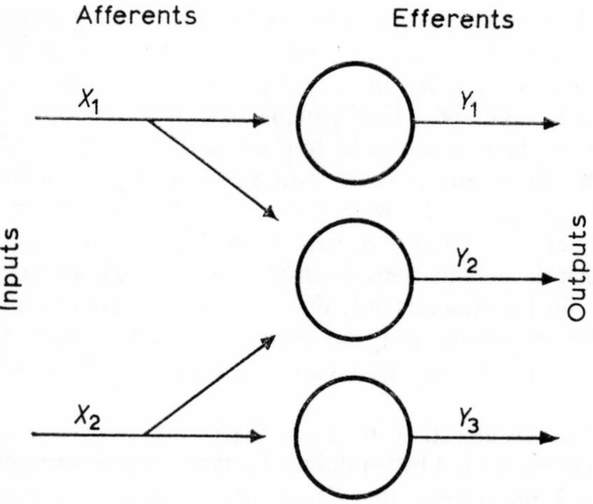

FIG. 69. Illustrating Uttley's (1954) classification machine.

inputs and outputs are digital. That is to say, a spatial pattern of inputs can either cause one signal of unit magnitude in any afferent conductor, X, or fail to set up such a signal. Thus, the afferent part of this simple classification system could only respond in three different ways to its environment, given by Table 3, where (1) indicates that an afferent

TABLE 3

	AFFERENT PATTERNS		
	I	*II*	*III*
Behaviour of X_1	1	0	1
Behaviour of X_2	0	1	1
Causing efferent signals from . . .	Y_1 Y_2	Y_2 Y_3	Y_1, Y_2 Y_3

signal was set up, and (0) implies that no signal was caused, within some short time interval δt. Provided that the efferent units, Y, can be excited by any single afferent signal, they will indicate unambiguously the nature of the input pattern in the manner listed in the last row of the table. As described, this system is only capable of classifying spatial patterns, composed of simultaneous inputs. Uttley points out that "... if spatio-temporal patterns are to be distinguished, each input signal must pass through a series of delays, after each of which a separate connexion is taken to the classification system". Thus, in addition to the three efferent units of Fig. 69, we should require at least two more indicators for X_1–before–X_2 and X_2–before–X_1.

Uttley's discussion of classification systems (1954) was intended to provide a mathematical analogue for the ways in which the central nervous system might classify incoming sensory information. Indeed, it is easy to see its relevance to Sherrington's concepts of spatial summation in the spinal cord, where the 'subliminal fringe' represents neurones of the class illustrated by Y_1 and Y_3 of Fig. 69. Again, in the visual cerebral cortex, there are neurones which respond predominately to excitation by the ipsilateral retina, those for which the contralateral retina is dominant and some which are most readily excited by simultaneous inputs from both retinae (see p. 165) (Burns, Heron & Grafstein, 1960; Hubel & Wiesel, 1962)—comparable to Y_1, Y_2 and Y_3 of Fig. 69. An even more striking parallel can be taken from the work of Hubel and Wiesel, who have recorded from single neurones of the cat and the monkey. When their results are combined with those of Kuffler (1953), who examined the properties of mammalian retinal ganglion cells, it becomes clear that the visual system operates as a classification machine. The output from many light receptors of the retina converges upon one retinal ganglion cell; there is a one-to-one correspondence between these ganglion cells and neurones in the lateral geniculate body (Hubel & Wiesel, 1961); but there is again convergence of fibres from the lateral geniculate upon individual nerve cells in the visual cerebral cortex (Hubel & Wiesel, 1962). Within the cerebral cortex, the output from one functional class of neurone appears to converge upon another functional class. At each stage in this series of repeated convergence of pathways, the type of retinal stimulus most likely to excite changes with the apparent 'purpose' of extracting certain information from any complex pattern of light upon the retina. Figure 70 is intended as a summary of the findings of Hubel and Wiesel and shows how the most exciting pattern on the retina changes as information is passed back along the central pathway of the visual system. At the receiving end of this system we find, in the visual cortex, cells which indicate the location and orientation of a line or border in the visual field. Hubel & Wiesel (1962) called them cells with simple receptive fields; one might also name them location-orientation

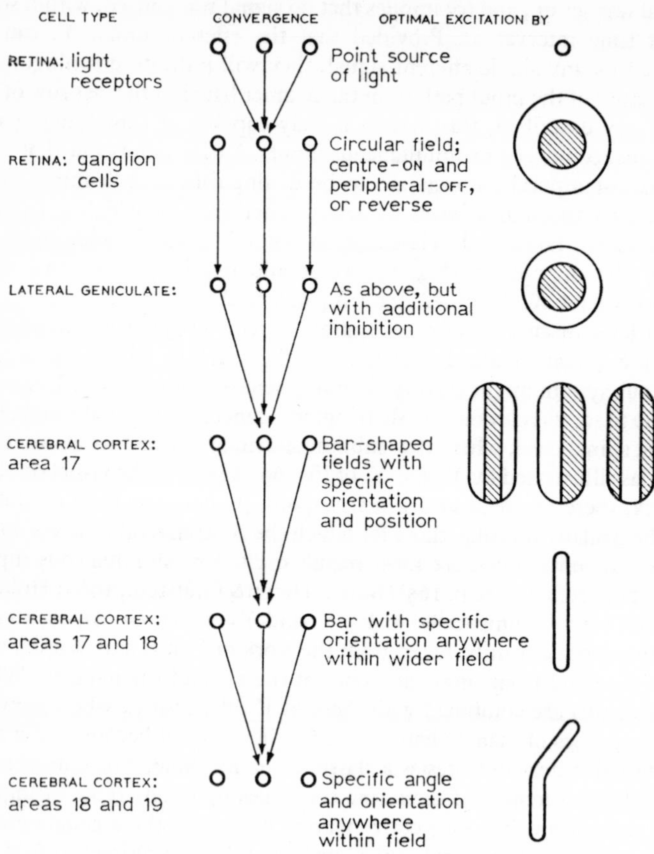

FIG. 70. A summary of the functional classes of neurone that have been described at various levels in the nervous system. See Hubel & Wiesel (1965*a*).

detectors. Then again in the cerebral cortex are orientation detectors (Hubel & Wiesel describe these as cells with complex fields) that are much less fussy about the exact location of a retinal border, provided that its orientation is correct. The last functional category of cortical cells identified by Hubel & Wiesel (1965*a*) (their cells with hypercomplex fields) might be classed as corner detectors.

Although a classification system usefully emulates some of the properties of a central nervous system, it cannot learn. 'The unit of a classification system returns after indicating to its original state; so because there are no stored after-effects, the behaviour of the system is unaffected by its past activity' (Uttley, 1956). In this sense, it belongs to the 'telephone exchange' class of analogue and cannot change its properties as the result of past experience.

One could construct a classification system with the necessary plasticity by the addition of new units capable of counting the number of times that X_1 and X_2 of Fig. 68 had fired during some past period time, T, both alone and simultaneously. Provided that the output of these new counting units was made to control the future conductivities of junctions between afferents and efferents, we should have a machine capable of changing its behaviour as a result of past experience. Uttley (1956) called this device a *conditional probability* machine.

At this point, it may be helpful to summarize and define a little more precisely the concepts and symbols that are used in this discussion of learning machines. The following notation applies to a system of afferent units, X, and efferent units, Y.

x and y = the frequencies of signals in X and Y respectively.
xy = the frequency with which X and Y fire simultaneously; i.e. within the same short time, δt.
$x \rightarrow y$ = the frequency with which a signal in X 'causes' one in Y; i.e. precedes one in Y by a short time, δt.
$\bar{x}y$ = the frequency of firing in Y not caused by signals in X; thus, $\bar{x}y = y - (x \rightarrow y)$.
$x_1 x_2$ = the frequency with which two afferent units, X_1 and X_2, fire simultaneously; i.e. within the same short time, δt.
$S(x)$ = the total count of past signals in X; a similar meaning attaches to $S(y)$, $S(xy)$, etc.
$S_{t-T}^{t}(x)$ = the total count of signals in X during the last T seconds.
C_{xy} = conductivity of the XY junction and is defined as the probability that a signal in X will cause one in Y; thus $C_{xy} = (x \rightarrow y)/x$.

We can now describe a conditional probability machine as a classification machine, with additional units capable of computing:

$$\frac{S(x_1 x_2)}{S(x_1)} \quad \text{and} \quad \frac{S(x_1 x_2)}{S(x_2)} \qquad \text{(see Fig. 68)}$$

Such a machine, in computing $S(x_1 x_2)/S(x_1)$, is estimating the probability of a signal in X_2, given that there is a simultaneous signal in X_1—the conditional probability of simultaneous signals in X_1 and X_2. Uttley has shown that many aspects of classical conditioned reflexes can be emulated by a conditional probability machine. Suppose that in Fig. 71 X_1 represents the afferent pathways excited by a conditioned stimulus, while X_2 represents afferents from the unconditioned stimulus. Then the table below records a sequence of signals, (1), as they might occur in

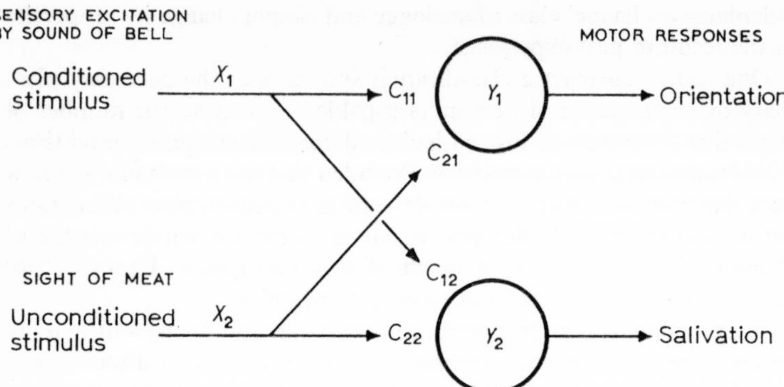

FIG. 71. The elements of a conditional probability machine necessary for learning.

X_1 and X_2; it also shows the values of $S(x_1x_2)/S(x_1)$ at three times during this sequence:

X_1	01010101	11111111	11111111	11111111
X_2	00110011	11111111	11111111	11111111
$\frac{S(x_1x_2)}{S(x_1)}$	$\frac{2}{4}$	$\frac{10}{12}$	$\frac{18}{20}$	$\frac{26}{28}$

Time has been divided into units of δt, chosen sufficiently small that not more than one afferent signal can occur in any one interval of δt. Four consecutive blocks of time of duration, $8 \times \delta t$ each, are shown in the table above. In the first block of this table, it is supposed that the excitations of X_1 and X_2 were statistically independent; in the remaining blocks of time, conditioned and unconditioned stimuli were presented together, causing simultaneous signals in X_1 and X_2. It will be seen that, as the joint presentations continue, the value of $S(x_1x_2)/S(x_1)$ rises and will approach unity asymptotically. Suppose now, that at the outset of this experiment C_{11} and C_{22} were very high, so that every signal in X_1 caused a signal in Y_1 and every signal in X_1 caused a signal from Y_2; in contrast, at the beginning of the experiment, C_{12} and C_{21} are assumed to be very low so that an extremely small fraction of signals in X_1 caused a response in Y_2 and signals of X_2 rarely caused a signal from Y_1. Then, provided the unit which computes $S(x_1x_2)/S(x_1)$ in the system controls the conductivity C_{12}, in such a way that C_{12} increases as $S(x_1x_2)/S(x_1)$ approaches unity, X_1 will become more and more likely to excite Y_2 as 'conditioning' proceeds. In this way the system behaves in a manner analogous to positive conditioning in the experimental animal. Uttley (1956) also shows how his conditional probability machine can stimulate the essential features of experimental extinction, external inhibition, reinforcement and differentiation (Pavlov, 1927).

The units for computing $S(x_1x_2)/S(x_1)$ and $S(x_1x_2)/S(x_2)$ are not shown in Fig. 71. These are units in a logical process and need not be represented by neurones in a nervous system. The required calculation could, in fact, be performed at the synaptic junctions between 'afferent' and 'efferent' neurones. C_{12} was defined as the probability that a signal in X_1 would cause a response in Y_2; it is, in fact, the instantaneous value of $(x_1 \rightarrow y_2)/x_1$. We have postulated that it varies in phase with the past history of X_1 and X_2, described by $S(x_1x_2)/S(x_1)$.

The term $S(x_1x_2)$ represents the total count of coincident signals in the afferents, X_1 and X_2. At first sight, it might appear that Uttley's conditional probability machine makes use of a parameter similar to presynaptic facilitation (Eccles, 1964) in biological nervous systems. It should be pointed out, however, that the nervous system could behave like a conditional probability machine without being dependent upon presynaptic influences. We have already assumed that nearly every signal in X_2 causes a response in Y_2. Therefore, we may write for the machine of Fig. 71:

$$C_{12} \propto \frac{S(x_1x_2)}{S(x_1)} \simeq \frac{S(x_1y_2)}{S(x_1)}$$

which would make conditioning dependent upon the relative times of firing of X_1 and Y_2—upon *trans*-synaptic events.

Unless we are to assume very different properties for the two junctions, X_1Y_2 and X_2Y_1, one would expect C_{21} to rise at the same time and for the same reason as C_{12}. Thus, after a period of conditioning as illustrated in the table above, one would expect to find that signals in X_2 had a high probability of exciting Y_1. This property is not consistent with the facts of experimental psychology. The analogous result in an animal conditioning experiment would be one in which, at the end of classical positive conditioning, the animal would behave as though it had heard a bell (and perhaps show an orientation response) whenever meat was presented. To take another example, although I salivate whenever I watch a lemon being sliced, I do not think of lemons whenever I salivate.

One way out of this difficulty, is to assume that the X_2 afferents of Fig. 71 are excited far more often than are the X_1 afferents. This would mean that $S(x_1x_2)/S(x_1)$ increased far more rapidly than did $S(x_1x_2)/S(x_1)$. However, this seems a somewhat unreasonable restriction to place on the operation of the conditional probability machine, in order to make it function in a more animal-like fashion.

It seems more likely that the failings of the machine referred to above are due to the fact that it does not take order of presentation of stimuli into account, although this factor is known to be vital in the formation of conditioned reflexes. Some small changes in the properties of this machine would make it behave in a more reasonable way. Suppose, for instance, that the conditioned and unconditioned stimuli set up signals in X_1 and X_2, the frequency of which declined progressively from a peak at the beginning of each stimulus, and that signals persist after the stimulation is over—in the manner of a biological after-discharge. The behaviour postulated is illustrated in Fig. 72. Suppose also that the

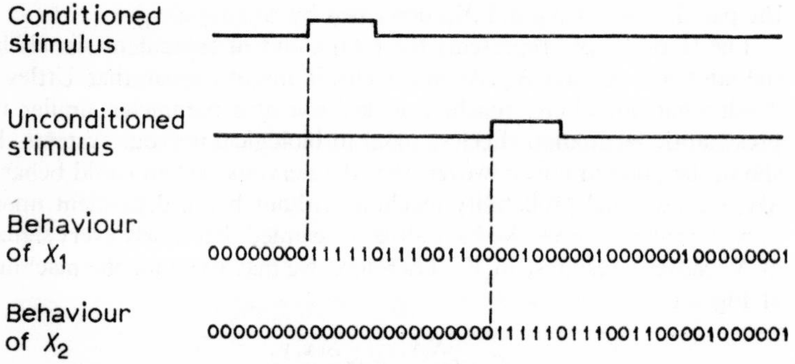

FIG. 72. Illustrating the way in which after-discharge might account for the dependence of conditioned reflex formation upon sequence of stimuli.

recent history of $S(x_1x_2)/S(x_1)$ determined the present value of C_{12}, so that:

$$C_{12} \propto \frac{S_{t-T}^{t}(x_1x_2)}{S_{t-T}^{t}(x_2)}$$

If T, the time for which the 'counters' of Uttley's conditional probability machine integrate past behaviour, is long by comparison with the duration of postulated after-discharge and the interval between presentations of stimuli, then C_{12} and C_{21} will change in the same way during conditioning, since in these circumstances:

$$\frac{S_{t-T}^{t}(x_1x_2)}{S_{t-T}^{t}(x_1)} = \frac{S_{t-T}^{t}(x_1x_2)}{S_{t-T}^{t}(x_2)}$$

However, if T is assumed shorter than the duration of after-discharges illustrated in Fig. 72,

$$C_{12} \propto \frac{S_{t-T}^{t}(x_1x_2)}{S_{t-T}^{t}(x_1)} > \frac{S_{t-T}^{t}(x_1x_2)}{S_{t-T}^{t}(x_2)} \propto C_{21}$$

Thus, essentially by adding the property that we have called after-discharge, Uttley's original conditional probability machine becomes more animal-like in its behaviour. It pays attention to the order in which afferent stimuli occur, and responds to repetition of a sequence of stimuli, S_1, S_2, in such a way that any original response to S_2 becomes ultimately a response to S_1 as well.

This discussion and development of Uttley's learning machine may be summarized by saying that a model with many properties of the mammalian central nervous system may be constructed from an assembly of units, each unit containing three model neurones so arranged that two afferent members, X_1 and X_2, converge upon one efferent member of the unit, Y. This, of course, is one way of describing a nerve net (see p. 58). Provided that spatial summation is possible at the interneural junctions of this system, it will operate as a crude classification machine. Provided that the present conductivity of all its junctions is governed by some rule of the form:

$$C_{x_1 y} \propto \frac{S^t_{t-T}(x_1 x_2)}{S^t_{t-x}(x_1)}$$

its present responses should depend upon past experience of its environment, in a manner that roughly emulates the behaviour of an intelligent animal.

The value of theoretical models

The fact that a conditional probability machine may fail to imitate some aspect of mammalian behaviour should not be allowed to diminish our respect for its usefulness. No model is perfect and the concept of conditional probability, like the other model nervous systems that have been examined during recent years, has at least introduced to neurophysiology new ways of thought and new hypotheses. On the other hand, brain modelling has often been criticized as a pastime; for this reason, it seems worthwhile to discuss briefly the value and disadvantages of model-learning systems.

Young (1964) claims that we do not understand a system until we are in a position to build a model of it. He says, "What answer do we expect when we ask, 'How does the brain work?' How should we know whether we had found the right answer? There is clearly some relation between this form of words and that of an engineer, who would say 'I know how it works' of a machine with the structure and connections of whose parts he was so familiar that he could take it to pieces and put it together again. Do we mean to imply that we should hope to be able to do this with a brain? I believe that in the last analysis this is the most useful criterion by which we should consider ourselves satisfied that we understand a living system." While this statement clearly contains an element of truth, it suggests that 'understanding' does not mean quite the same to an anatomist as to a physiologist. I am sure that any methodical historian or philosopher could dismantle my car and reassemble it, provided that he took careful notes, listing the original position of each component. But this tedious operation would bring him no nearer to understanding the principles of internal combustion. Clearly, a model cannot, and is not expected to, emulate all the properties of the brain; nor need it be a tangible construction of moving parts or of electronic components—it could be no more than a series of mathematical equations. It should, however, be a system constructed of parts with which the builder is 'familiar', understanding at the same time the contribution made by each part to the function of the whole.

Nevertheless, the real value of a model does not lie in its ability to imitate nature. A useful model employs certain hypotheses in order to make predictions that would be tedious or impossible in its absence. It can be valuable for exactly the same reason that an analogue computer has value when programmed to emulate some of the known properties of a biological system. Such analogue computation is useless unless employed to test some theory. The computer may be supplied with certain properties of the system to be copied, and programmed also with one or more hypothetical properties. If the result is the prediction of an additional property which was either known to be true, or is later found to be true, some justification for the hypotheses is provided. The prediction of properties that do not correspond with observation will likewise weaken belief in the hypotheses. It is in this sense that a model is most useful. Thus, a model does not have merit because it behaves like a brain. If it was a well-designed model, this would be the least that we should expect from it. It becomes useful only when it behaves more like a brain than was apparently dictated by its original specifications.

These considerations do not provide much justification for the building of electronic tortoises and the like. Nevertheless, it has to be admitted that the creation of such scientific toys has served at least one purpose. Ashby's homeostat (1952) and Grey Walter's goal-seeking artificial tortoise (1953) produced an intriguing advertisement for the usefulness of cybernetic concepts in neurophysiological thought. Seeing contributes towards believing, even for the best trained minds.

There are two ways in which models can prove useful. First, they necessarily force the biologist to define his concepts clearly, for one cannot build a working model or a mathematical equation from ill-defined components. There can be little doubt that contemporary neurophysiological thought is often hampered by the use of terms with uncertain meaning. To be convinced of this one has only to consider the frequent usage of words such as fatigue, accommodation, habituation and refractory; or again, words such as potentiation, augmentation and facilitation. Not only can model building help to define relevant concepts, but it can also provide quantitative and mathematical relations between these concepts which may later be tested and used. Thus model building has the advantage of forcing the biologist to be a little more precise in his thinking and to make his observations more quantitative.

Considered in this way, Uttley's examination of the properties of conditional probability computers has proved an invaluable contribution to the study of learning in animals. The success or failure of these machines in copying animal behaviour is a minor part of their scientific usefulness; indeed, in the preceding pages, some failings of the original conditional probability machine have been pointed out. Uttley's work has indicated types of change that *may* occur at the synaptic junctions between nerve cells, that *could* explain some aspects of simple learning. The result is a number of hypotheses which can be tested. For instance, do synapses become more conducting, the more often they have transmitted excitation in the past? We have already pointed out that the successful emulation of some aspects of animal learning by conditional probability machines depends upon the incorporation of 'synaptic junctions' whose conductivity rises as the result of what looks like some form of presynaptic facilitation. Is there in fact physiological evidence for changes of this nature?

Evidence for prolonged changes of synaptic conductance in the c.n.s.

In order to test this or any other hypothesis concerning long-lasting changes of synaptic conductance in the central nervous system, one must first find a site at which such changes occur and then devise a preparation suitable for measurement of the relevant factors. Relatively persistent changes in the conductivity of junctions in the spinal cord have been described by Lloyd (1949) and by Eccles & McIntyre (1953). There are good reasons, however, to look for the conductivity changes that may underlie simple learning in the mammalian cerebral cortex (Burns, 1958), and consequently it seems sensible to ask whether records of electrical activity of the cortex ever demonstrate 'persistent' changes as a result of past sensory input.

Evidence from gross electrodes

There has been evidence for some time that the proper sequence of sensory stimuli can produce long-lasting changes in the electroencephalogram or electrocorticogram. In the early 1930's, Durup and Fessard were using a camera to photograph the disappearance of human alpha rhythm in response to light. They reported (1935) that the click of their camera shutter soon acquired the properties of the light-stimulus and would produce the same electrographic response, even when the light was withheld. They were able to show that this auditory stimulus acquired new properties because of its repeated past association in time with visual excitation. Repetition of the clicks alone did not induce the response, but would produce the extinction of an already existing response.

This observation formed the basis of many subsequent attempts to 'condition the electroencephalogram'. For instance, Jasper & Shagass (1941*a*, *b*), using the reduction of alpha rhythm as a response, were able to demonstrate nearly all forms of Pavlovian conditioning including trace and delayed reflexes. They said, "The alpha block conditioned to sound or time . . . is, however, very unstable: appearing with relatively little practice and showing rapid extinction. In some experiments extinction occurred after as few as three conditioned responses." Morrel & Jasper (1956) found that during the early stages of visual conditioning, tone or touch used as conditioned stimulus produced a widespread desynchronization in all cortical areas; later during the learning process the electroencephalographic response to the conditioned stimulus was restricted to the visual region. Morrel (1961) has reviewed the literature concerned with this subject and summarizes the situation by saying: "since as a result of the experimental procedure an acoustic stimulus produces an electric response (local visual cortex desynchronization) which was not previously in its repertory, loses it if reinforcement is omitted (extinction), regains it when pairing is resumed and since another stimulus which was not reinforced does not produce the response, it seems reasonable to describe this as conditioning. What is conditioned, however, is not a particular electrical configuration but its topographical distribution."

It is quite clear that changes can be produced in the electroencephalogram by procedures that are similar to those used when setting up a conditioned reflex in an experimental animal. Unfortunately, however, the nature of these changes is not easy to analyse because at present the meaning of the electrocorticogram in terms of cellular activity is itself unknown. For the same reason, experiments in which the cortical response evoked by sensory excitation is altered by conditioning procedures (Jouvet & Hernandez-Peon, 1957) are not likely to be informative about the underlying mechanisms of memory formation.

Evidence from extracellular micro-electrodes

More encouraging in this respect are experiments in which the behaviour of single cortical neurones is studied during the establishment of a conditioned reflex. Jasper, Ricci & Doane (1961) have described the behaviour of single cells in the monkey's motor cortex during avoidance conditioning, but concluded that it was necessary to look outside the motor cortex in order to find evidence of the change of pathways that must underlie conditioning.

There are two reliable ways of producing a long-lasting change in the behaviour of cortical units. In the undisturbed brain, the mean frequency of discharge of cortical nerve cells per minute remains constant for many hours, but this mean frequency can be reset to a new constant value by a relatively short period of either subcortical stimulation or unit polarization. Figure 73 shows the changes in mean frequency of a

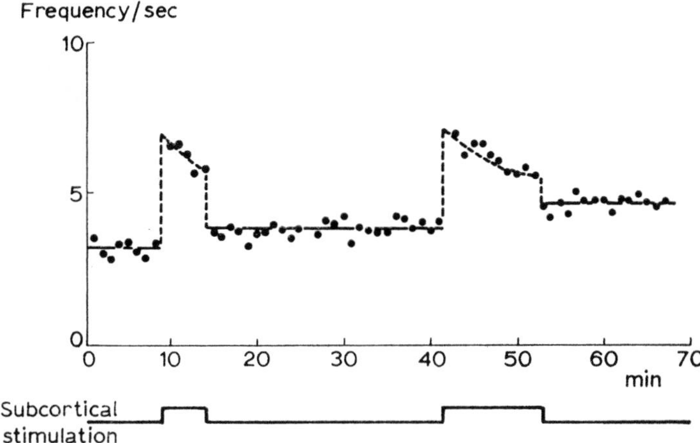

FIG. 73. Showing the immediate effects and after-effects of periods of 5 and 10 minutes' subcortical stimulation, at 10/sec, upon the frequency of discharge of a cortical neurone (calculated from count in 60 sec). Stimuli =0·25 msec duration. The continuous horizontal lines represent the arithmetic means of the points through which they are drawn. (The pre- and post-stimulation means are significantly different: $p < 0.01$.) The same neurone as in Fig. 74.

cortical neurone, produced by a 5-minute, and later by a 10-minute period of subcortical stimulation at 10/sec. The experiment was performed in the isolated forebrain of the unanaesthetized cat; the recorded unit was in the suprasylvian gyrus. The conditioning stimuli, given through fine wire electrodes thrust into the white matter just below the recorded cell, reset the frequency of spontaneous activity to a new value which was maintained without significant drift for a period of 25 minutes. Bindman, Lippold & Redfearn (1964), recording from cortical units in the anaesthetized rat, have produced similar long-lasting changes of mean frequency with short periods of surface polarization. The after-effect of conditioning procedures persisted without attenuation for more than an hour. Persistent changes in unit frequency can also be produced by polarizing current which is restricted to the vicinity of the recorded cell. This can be done by passing a steady current through the same micropipette that is employed for recording unit discharge (Bindman, Lippold & Redfearn, 1964); because spikes can be recorded through an RC-coupling of short time constant, the recorded activity is only interrupted for a few milliseconds at the ON and OFF of the polarizing current. Figure 74 shows the effect upon a cortical unit

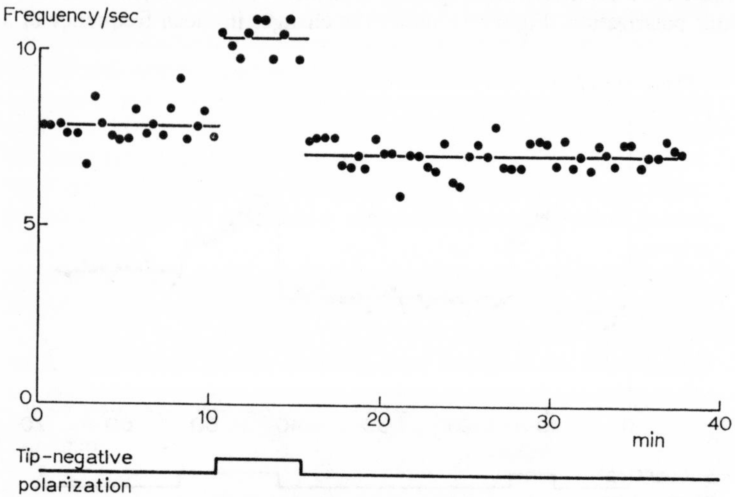

FIG. 74. Showing the immediate effect and after-effect of 5 minutes of tip-negative polarization upon the frequency of discharge of a cortical neurone (frequency calculated from count/30 sec). Internal diameter of micropipette used for both recording and polarization was 3 μ; polarizing current = 0·3 μA. Horizontal lines represent the arithmetic means of the points through which they are drawn. (Difference between pre- and post-polarization means is statistically significant; Fisher's *t* test gives $p < 0.01$. The same neurone as in Fig. 73.

(the same as that providing Fig. 73) of a 5-minute period of tip-negative polarization with 0·3 $\mu A/30\mu^2$. The internal diameter of the micro-electrode's tip was about 3 μ.

There seems no doubt that long-lasting changes in the behaviour of cortical cells can be affected by such procedures. If one assumes that the 'spontaneous' discharge of cortical neurones is the result of their excitation by other central neurones (see p. 74), then an alteration of mean frequency probably implies a persistent change in the conductivity of those synapses that link the recorded neurone with neighbouring cells.

Although experiments of this sort are easy to perform, it is not possible to find an unequivocal interpretation of their results. One tenable explanation of Figs. 73 and 74 might run as follows:

1. Mean frequency was immediately increased by tip-negative polarization, because this brought about a reduction of membrane potential,

which made the recorded unit more responsive to a constant input of excitation from its neighbours (Frank & Fuortes, 1956; Coombs, Curtis & Eccles, 1957). The polarizing current used in this experiment was not sufficient to drive the cell directly.

2. This temporary increase of traffic across the unit's synaptic junctions was itself the cause of a long-lasting decrease in conductivity of those same junctions; on this view, the latter would be responsible for the observed persistent decrease in mean firing rate that followed polarization.
3. Subcortical stimulation, which also produced an immediate increase frequency, did so by driving the cell through a small fraction of those synaptic connections responsible for its spontaneous activity.
4. Therefore, during conditioning stimulation, there would have been post-synaptic activity without corresponding presynaptic action at the majority of synapses.
5. This period of increased post-synaptic activity could have been responsible for facilitation at those synapses, leading to the observed persistent rise in mean frequency of discharge which followed conditioning stimulation.

This picture of events would imply that an increase of $\bar{x}y$ (using the symbols of p. 145) brought about a rise in conductivity. It would also suggest that an increase in usage of a synaptic pathway (temporary increase of $(x \rightarrow y)$) caused a decrease in synaptic conductivity—an interpretation that conflicts with popular belief.

The direct measurement of synaptic resistance

The argument above is not particularly convincing. It necessarily makes reasonable but untested assumptions about the distribution and action of polarizing current, in an attempt to deduce, by indirect means, the nature of changes in synaptic conductivity. Moreover, such experiments depend upon measurement of mean discharge frequency, a parameter of unit behaviour which one would expect to be relatively insensitive to functional changes (see p. 118). Contemporary averaging techniques make possible a relatively direct measurement of synaptic conductivity and thus enable one to find out which aspects, if any, of the past behaviour of two neurones determine the present conductivity of the synapses between them. The experiments described below are incomplete. My excuse for presenting a brief account of unfinished work is that I believe it demonstrates the usefulness of a particular technique and line of argument.

A cortical unit which receives excitation from electrodes in the white matter immediately below, will usually show in the post-stimulus histogram a clear-cut response of short latency (Fig. 75). The conductivity of the *system* can be defined for practical purposes as:

$$C = \frac{\text{Area of response in the P.S.H.}}{\text{Number of subcortical stimuli provided}}$$

a definition which is consistent with that given earlier on p. 145. Changes in conductivity can, of course, only be measured if the stimulus is not maximal with respect to the recorded unit and occasionally fails to drive the cell. The system considered would include axons excited by the subcortical-stimulating electrodes, the recorded unit and any interneurones there may be between these two. In the case of short-latency responses, as in Fig. 75a, one can be sure that not more than one inter-

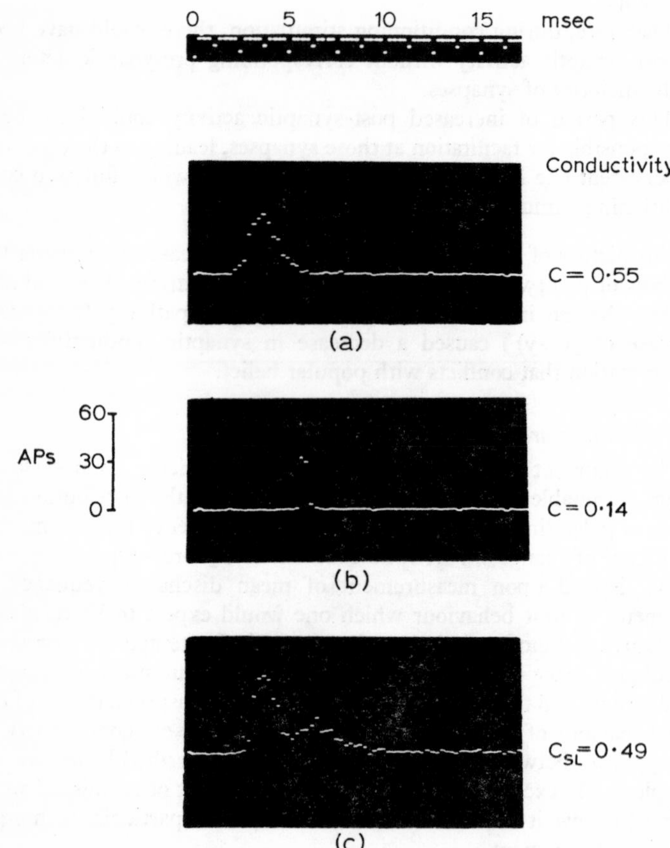

FIG. 75. Various post-stimulus histograms obtained from different cells in isolated cerebral cortex.
(From Bliss, Burns & Uttley, 1968, in preparation.)

neurone is involved, implying not more than two synapses between input and output. Sometimes, however, responses have longer latency (Fig. 75b), or they may be diphasic as in Fig. 75c. In the latter case, the second phase of the response indicates either excitation that has travelled by a longer route than was responsible for the first phase, or that the cell has been fired twice in response to excitation through only one path. This last possibility is almost always excluded by finding that the cell often fires in the second phase only; thus, experiments providing diphasic responses frequently give information about conductivity in two parallel pathways simultaneously.

In order to study the effects upon present conductivity of past behaviour of the inputs and outputs of the system, it is important to maintain control of spontaneous activity. This is most conveniently affected by working in slabs of neurologically isolated cerebral cortex, where spontaneous activity is absent. For this reason, we (Bliss, Burns & Uttley, 1968) arranged to record from a unit which could be excited by either of the two pathways illustrated in Fig. 76. It is important to stress that the arrows of this figure do not represent individual axons, but indicate routes, which may consist of several neurones providing a functional connection between stimulating electrodes and recorded unit. Thus, X_1 of this figure indicates the functional pathway from a non-polarizable stimulating electrode, resting lightly on the brain's surface, to the recorded cell; X_2 indicates the neural connection between a non-polarizable subcortical-stimulating electrode and the recorded neurone. With this arrangement, it is possible to make continuous measurements of the conductivity, C_{X_2Y}, between X_2 and Y, by giving submaximal test stimuli once a second through the stimulating electrodes, S_2. (C_{X_1Y} can be measured in a similar way.) It proved more convenient to use standard bursts of test stimuli—say, 5 stimuli repeated at 30/sec—than to use single stimuli. Most cortical units respond more controllably to this treatment and the procedure also allows one to use temporal summation to vary the probability of X_2 exciting Y. While measuring conductivity in this way, with standard bursts of test stimuli, we have been able to change x, y and $(x \rightarrow y)$ for short conditioning periods and observe the subsequent changes in C_{X_2Y}.

If, for example, we wished to study such changes of conductivity in the pathway X_2Y of Fig. 76 in response to short periods of increase in x, y and $(x \rightarrow y)$, we would condition the system with 5-minute periods of:

1. *Increase in* x *alone* The test stimulus strength and frequency within the burst would be so adjusted that, while the test burst produced a submaximal response, additional stimuli of the same strength but lower frequency produced none. We could then increase x for a period without producing additional responses from Y.

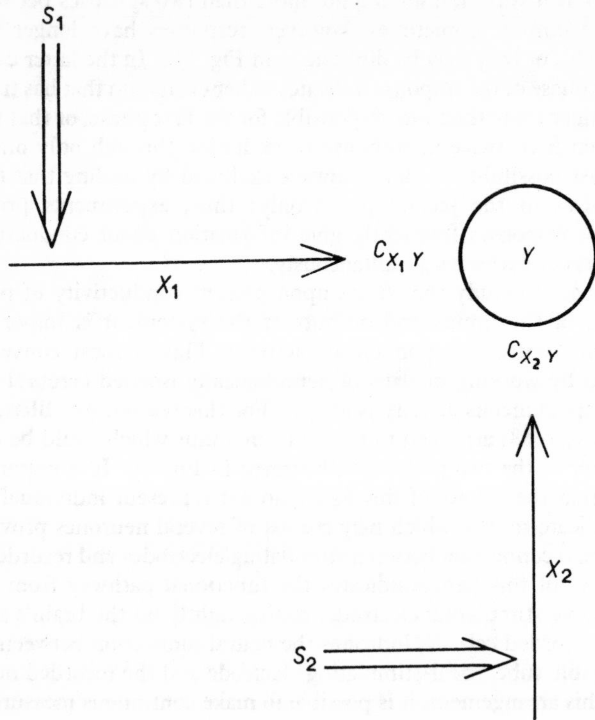

FIG. 76. Illustrating pathways in isolated cerebral cortex through which cortical units, Y can be excited. X_1 represents a transcortical pathway that can be excited through stimulation, S_1, of the pial surface. X_2 indicates a pathway originating in the subcortical white matter that can be excited by a subcortical stimulus (S_2).

2. *Increase of* y *alone* A period of excitation of the recorded unit through the pathway $X_1 Y$ provided this.
3. *Increase of* (x→y) The test stimulus strength and frequency within the burst would be so adjusted that a decrease in the interval between individual stimuli of the burst produced an increased frequency of firing from Y. In this way, we could temporarily increase $(x \rightarrow y)$ without increasing x. (This procedure necessarily produced a concomitant increase of y).

Figure 77 illustrates the results of procedure (2) above.

The main purpose of these experiments was to determine the signs of the coefficients a, b and c in an equation of the form:

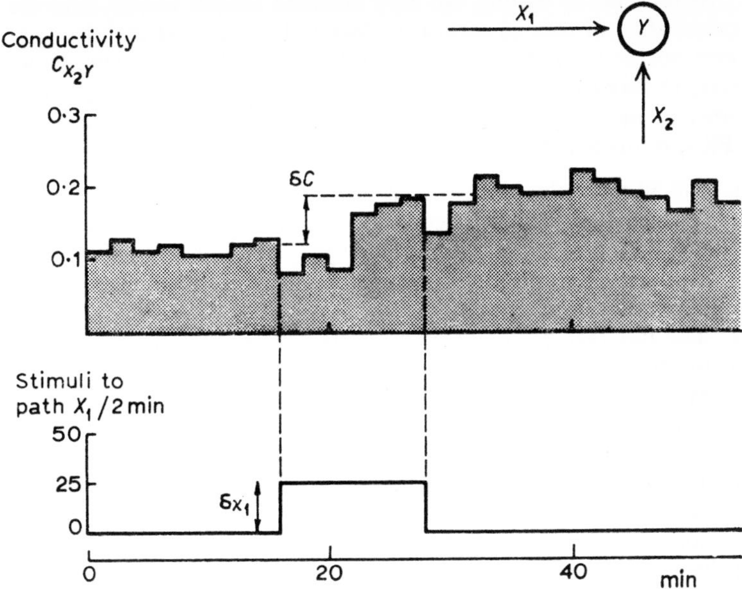

FIG. 77. The change in conductivity through a subcortical pathway, X_2 produced by a 12-min period of excitation of a transcortical pathway, X_1. Isolated cerebral cortex. Test stimuli (consisting of bursts of 6 stimuli at 50/sec, repeated every 12 sec) were delivered to the subcortical white matter. The surface stimuli used for conditioning produced multiple responses from the recorded unit, Y, and increased the rate of discharge of Y per minute some ten-fold during the conditioning period. (From Bliss, Burns & Uttley, 1968, in preparation.)

$$\delta C = f[a.\delta x, b.\delta y, c.\delta(x \rightarrow y)]$$

where δx is defined as the immediate alteration in x during the conditioning period,

δC is the change in conductivity produced by this conditioning period, as indicated in Fig. 77.

and the definitions of δy and $\delta(x \rightarrow y)$ are similar to that for δx above. It should, perhaps, be said once more that any relationship between the parameters listed above is only a statement about the behaviours of input and output of a system containing an uncertain number of neurones and types of synapse. Strictly speaking, C is only a measure of conductivity through the system, under constant conditions. Only by making the unwarranted assumption that all cortical synapses are functionally similar, could one use this parameter as a measure of the conductivity of a cortical synapse.

At the time of writing, we have obtained reliable results from the examination of only 26 cortical pathways. In 9 of these pathways, we were unable to produce any detectable change of conductivity. However, 17 pathways exhibited a change of conductivity following one or other of the conditioning manoeuvres listed above. Our conclusions (Bliss, Burns & Uttley, 1968) from this work run as follows:

1. Not all the pathways investigated have shown persistent changes in C which, like that illustrated in Fig. 77, exhibited no sign of attenuation during 20 minutes or so. Some 30% have shown an after-effect in which C returned to its preconditioning level with a time constant of roughly 10 minutes.
2. The fact that persistent after-effects can be observed in slabs of isolated cerebral cortex implies that the changes illustrated in Figs. 73 and 74 can have a cortical origin. It becomes clear that there must be cortical synaptic junctions, the conductivity of which is plastic and depends upon the past behaviour of the neurones which they link.
3. The conductivity of the junction between two nerve cells, X and Y, can only be predicted from a knowledge of their past relative frequencies of discharge.
4. Persistent changes in conductivity were usually correlated negatively with temporary changes in (x), negatively with temporary changes in $(x \rightarrow y)$, and positively with temporary changes in (y).
5. Thirteen of the 17 pathways for which conditioning procedures caused a change of δC, showed properties consistent with the formula:

$$k \,.\, \delta C = a \,.\, \frac{\delta x}{x} + b \,.\, \frac{\delta y}{y} + c \,.\, \frac{\delta(x \rightarrow y)}{(x \rightarrow y)}$$

where k is a positive coefficient, which is usually different for each experiment and a, b and c are constants, such that a and c are negative, while b is positive.

These conclusions are particularly interesting in two respects. They provide little support for the existence of the 'practice-makes-perfect' type of cortical synapse—one which the more often it transmits activity, the more likely is it to do so in future. On the contrary, it appears that most cortical pathways are less likely to transmit information, the more often they are used. Thus, if the majority of cortical synapses obeyed a rule of the form described in (5) above, we should have a ready explanation of the surprising stability of discharge frequency per minute observed among cortical neurones.

This investigation of factors determining conductivity through pathways of cortical neurones was undertaken because of an interest in the physiology of learning. It has already established that relatively long-lasting changes in the conductivity of cortical synapses can occur; moreover, it has shown that the nature of changes in conductivity within the cortical grey matter can be predicted from a knowledge of the past history of inputs to, and outputs from, the cells considered. Nevertheless, one cannot be sure without further proof that the long-lasting changes in conductivity observed in such experiments are an essential component of the mechanism of simple learning. Further information of a different type will be required before this working hypothesis can become respectable. If the conductivity changes described above have anything to do with persistent and acquired changes of behaviour in the intact animal, one would expect them to be affected by those procedures that are known to affect learning. I am thinking here of Leao's spreading cortical depression (Bures & Buresova, 1956; Burns, 1958), and of light general anaesthesia (Summerfield & Steinberg, 1957; Robson, Burns & Welt, 1960). Then again, if further experimental results establish the formula of (5) above as a reliable and general statement, it will still be unclear how a nervous system, built of conducting units with these properties, could store and make future use of new sensory information.

CHAPTER 8

THE NEXT STEP

UNTIL some twenty years ago, attempts to explain function in the intact nervous system were necessarily dependent upon the results of experiments employing relatively large stimulating and recording electrodes. The only quantitative input-output relationships available to those who wished to build an interpretation of normal behaviour were relations between highly unphysiological stimuli and the consequent abnormal responses. While gross electrodes might record the synchronous discharge of many neighbouring neurones, they were incapable of registering the spatial and temporal detail of asynchronous activity. As a result, the physiologist unwittingly left his readers with an impression that central neurones only discharged when instructed to do so by a neurophysiologist—the system appeared to be an immense assembly of wholly predictable relationships.

The widespread, recent use of micro-electrodes has done much to alter this picture. One is now forced to think of most, if not all, central neurones as continually active; chattering away to one another ceaselessly, even when the animal is apparently doing nothing. Indeed, it is this continual activity on the part of 'unstimulated' central nerve cells which has forced the neurophysiologist to develop techniques of statistical averaging, so that responses to controlled physiological stimuli may be separated from noise.

The preceding chapters have largely been concerned with an assessment of the contribution made by statistical techniques to an understanding of the function in the normal animal. There seems no doubt that development of the micro-electrode and the use of electronic computers have considerably altered our qualitative picture of the nervous system. These relatively new techniques have made possible new experiments, and a new language in which to describe the behaviour of central neurones. But novelty is not necessarily progress; nor are these the only new techniques and languages available to neurophysiology. In the following paragraphs I shall try to summarize what I believe to be the present significant achievements of statistical neurophysiology, with the intention of later stressing the limitations of this method. Moreover, in order to maintain some sort of perspective, it seems important to close with some reference, however brief, to other equally promising lines of research and thought.

SUMMARY OF PRECEDING CHAPTERS

A number of relatively important concepts has emerged from the discussion on preceding pages. About some points it is possible to be fairly dogmatic; others suggest generalizations which, although not fully established, may serve as useful working hypotheses that could guide future investigation. Thus, the statements in my summary of the present achievements of statistical neurophysiology are not all of equal value. Perhaps the following list should be regarded as a number of generalizations about cortical neurones for which at least some support has been provided.

1. Most, if not all, neurones in the 'resting', unanaesthetized nervous system are continually active, displaying a constant mean frequency of discharge per minute, although the precise times of discharge are not predictable.
2. Mean frequency of discharge is an aspect of neural behaviour that is unlikely to be of great neurophysiological importance, since physiological stimuli produce a temporal redistribution of action potentials, often without significant alteration of mean frequency.
3. The response of neurones to constant physiological stimuli is stochastic in nature. Consequently, any meaningful relation between stimulus and unit response must be stated in terms of probability of discharge.
4. A physiological stimulus probably causes the same response in at least 100 'redundant' neurones, since identification of a simple test stimulus from records of a single unit often requires computation of the average response to about 100 identical stimuli.
5. The behaviour of cortical neurones is most readily disturbed by change of sensory input, causing bursts of action potentials, in a close-packed group of cortical afferents.
6. An effective stimulus produces a maximum difference between the firing rates of neighbouring cortical units, exciting some and depressing the activity of others.
7. In the presence of sensory stimulation, the nervous system appears to be stable when maximal disturbance of cortical neurones is restricted to the smallest possible number of neighbouring cortical elements.
8. Statistical techniques have provided a method for measuring the conductivity of cortical synapses, and suggest that the more often a synaptic pathway is used, the less conducting it becomes.

Whatever the future success of unit recordings made with extracellular micro-electrodes, the technique has certain obvious limitations. It only provides reliable information concerning the precise times of neuronal discharge. Records made in this way do not readily tell one why a unit fired, since physiological presynaptic events are not usually recorded. The extracellular micro-electrode does not give reliable information about any post-synaptic events that may precede discharge. Intracellular recordings would be more informative in this respect, but require a degree of mechanical stability that makes it difficult or impossible to watch the history of a single unit over many hours.

Moreover, records from a single neurone, whether made with an intra- or extracellular micro-electrode, offer only indirect information about the spatial spread of excitation among a population of neurones. The visual position plots referred to on p. 92 provide one example of an attempt to assess the distribution of excitation from observation of only one point in a cell network. It is, in fact, possible to obtain quite long records from several cortical units simultaneously, using a number of independent extracellular recording electrodes (Amassian, Berlin, Macy & Waller, 1959; Holmes & Houchin, 1966). Such multiple recordings could provide more direct information about the spatial spread of excitation. Indeed, if spatial and temporal patterns of activity within the nervous system determine its output, then cross-correlation of the times of discharge of separate neurones should provide some indication of the neural codes that underlie behaviour.

PROMISING ALTERNATIVE TECHNIQUES

The interdependence of the various parts of the mammalian central nervous system puts the neurophysiologist in nearly the same position as the astonomer—he can observe, but he may not meddle with the system. The neurophysiologist can only interfere with the brain in a very limited way if he is to preserve its function. Consequently, he has often been forced to use indirect methods and complicated apparatus to answer simple questions. The electroencephalographer justifies the use of sixteen simultaneous channels of record by reference to the complexity of the organ that he studies. Likewise, the neurophysiologist (once defined as an electroencephalographer with only two channels!) might now argue that the statistical treatment of data obtained from the mammalian nervous system is necessitated by its size and complexity. For these reasons, the study of simpler nervous systems is attractive; for one hopes that the rules of behaviour in simpler systems may be applicable, perhaps in modified form, to the working of the intact mammalian brain. In this connection, one might list three recent lines of investigation, each illustrative of an attempt to study a system of neurones that is simpler than that in the adult mammal—functional development of the immature mammalian nervous system, the nervous systems of other species and the study of neural tissue cultures.

Development of the nervous system

Hubel & Wiesel have recently turned their attention to questions concerning the development of the immature, mammalian visual system (Wiesel & Hubel, 1963, 1965*a*, *b*; Hubel & Wiesel, 1965*b*). They have tried to discover what factors determine the establishment and maintenance of functional connections between the retina and neurones of the visual cerebral cortex in kittens. In the mature animal, the majority of units in the visual cortex can be driven by appropriately placed changes of light intensity on either left or right retina, but it is usual for one or other retina to dominate (Hubel & Wiesel, 1962; Burns & Pritchard, 1967). Hubel and Wiesel devised a semi-quantitative method for classifying the retinal control of the cortical units that they studied. These neurones were classed into 7 groups, ranging from those driven by the contralateral retina only (Group 1), through those driven by both retinae equally (Group 4), to units that responded only to excitation of the ipsilateral retina (Group 7). Figure 78*a* shows the distribution within these groups of 223 cells tested in normal adult cats. It can be seen that the majority of cells can be driven from either retina, while the largest groups contain those cells that are almost equally controlled by either eye. The neural connections necessary to this distribution of ocular dominance must be formed at birth or soon afterwards, since Hubel & Wiesel (1963*b*) obtained results from 8 to 16-day-old kittens that were "... strikingly similar to those of adult cats."

If, during the first two months of life, pattern vision is prevented in one eye, either by sewing the lids together or with a translucent covering for that eye, the uncovered retina becomes dominant and few cells can be excited through the treated eye (Wiesel & Hubel, 1963*b*). It must be remembered that mobile, patterned light falling upon the uncovered retina will provide an effective control of the behaviour of cortical cells, while one would expect the absence of light or diffuse light upon the covered retina to be almost equally poor forms of cortical stimulation (Burns, Heron & Pritchard, 1962). One might therefore conclude that, during the early development of the nervous system, some aspect of the use of synapses caused them to maintain a low resistance; but subsequent results have shown the explanation to be more complex.

The pathological ocular dominance described in the preceding paragraph was found to be irreversible. Recovery periods up to one year following early monocular visual deprivation did not restore normal ocular dominance (Wiesel & Hubel 1965*b*). More interesting still, Hubel and Wiesel found that the distribution of dominance was normal in

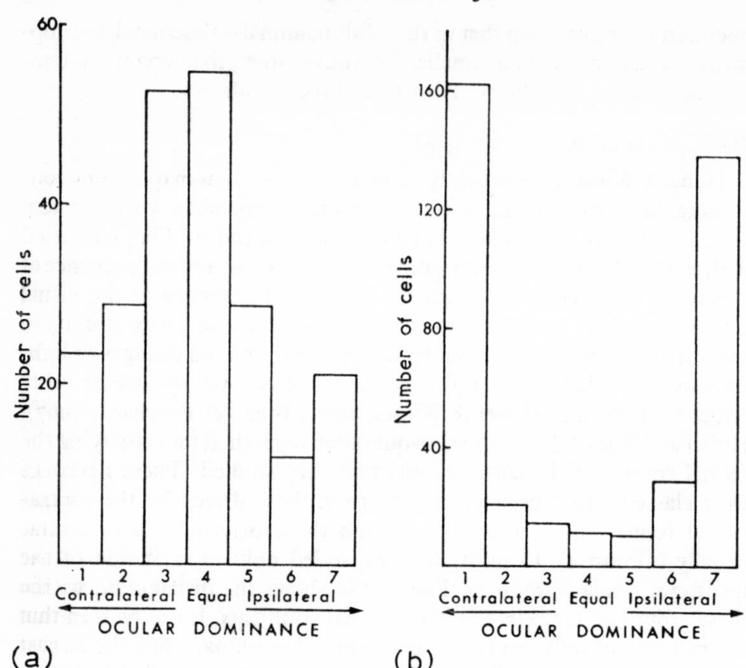

FIG. 78

(*a*) Ocular dominance of 223 cells recorded from a series of normal adult cats.

(*b*) Ocular dominance of 384 cells recorded from all four strabismus experiments.

(From (*a*) Hubel & Wiesel, 1962, *J. Physiol.*, 160, 106, Fig. 12; (*b*) Hubel & Wiesel, 1965*b*, *J. Neurophysiol.*, **28**, 1041, Fig. 5.)

kittens which had been prevented from using both eyes. This finding suggested that the degeneration of normal distribution which follows monocular deprivation might be caused by the absence of synchronous excitation (or inhibition) of cortical neurones by left and right eyes, a concept which was supported by the results of a most elegant set of experiments performed on young animals given an artificial squint (Hubel & Wiesel, 1965*b*). When the two eyes are properly aligned for normal binocular fusion, one presumes that every neurone in the optic cortex is influenced in a similar manner by changes in the light falling on anatomically corresponding districts of the two retinae. In the presence of strabismus, this cannot be so; a point source of light in the visual field will not cast images upon corresponding points of the two retinae and consequently cortical units can rarely receive comparable inputs from both eyes at the same time. Hubel and Wiesel showed that, after such treatment, few cortical neurones are equally excitable from either retina; the great majority of units is dominated by either the ipsilateral or the contralateral retina (Fig. 78*b*).

At first sight, these results stand in complete disagreement with those described in the preceding chapter. They suggest that where there are two inputs, X_1 and X_2, to a cortical neurone, Y, (see Fig. 68, p.141) the conductivity of the X_1Y synapse will become reduced if Y is persistently excited by X_2 alone. In the terminology of p. 145, they imply that changes in conductivity are negatively correlated with

$$\bar{x}y = y - (x \rightarrow y)$$

It must be remembered, however, that these are statements about the immature nervous system—one in which the number of synaptic connections between neurones is still variable. It is not unlikely that the rules governing the development of new pathways—the growth and maintenance of anatomical connections—are not the same as the rules dictating the resistance within these pathways, once they are firmly established. Indeed, Hubel and Wiesel have found that those experimental procedures that disturb the development of normal ocular dominance in newborn kittens are without effect upon adult animals (Wiesel & Hubel, 1963*b*).

These first results of a new experimental method that I have outlined above may or may not ultimately prove relevant to an understanding of learning mechanisms. In either case they describe a clear-cut and readily controllable plasticity of the central nervous system. Enough has probably been said to illustrate the power of this technique and to indicate its promise for the future.

Simpler nervous systems

The anatomical arrangement of the central nervous system in cephalopods is quite different from that in vertebrates. This is scarcely surprising since the philogenetic development of these two organs has proceeded along quite independent lines for some 500 million years. Nevertheless, similar conditioned reflexes can be established in both dog and octopus, and the latter often learns faster. It was this fact, among others, that led Young and his collaborators to begin a thorough investigation of the learning in cephalopods (Young, 1964). It seemed as though exploration of the similar behaviour of two systems that were so different in gross structure might reveal those factors at the cellular level that were responsible for all learning. This objective has not yet been realized, although the work has undoubtedly proved rewarding in many other ways. A long series of experiments has at least established that, while the cephalopod nervous system is very different from that in vertebrates, it is quite as complex.

An alternative approach to comparative neurophysiology is based upon the assumption that species showing different overall behaviour may nevertheless be governed by similar central mechanisms. This belief forms part of the justification for investigating relatively small neural networks in much simpler animals than the cat or monkey. The recent work of Kandel and Tauc provides an excellent illustration of this type of investigation (Kandel & Tauc, 1964; 1965*a*, *b*; Tauc, 1965; Kandel, Frazier & Coggershall, 1966).

They have investigated heterosynaptic facilitation in the abdominal ganglia of sea-slugs (*Aplysia depilans*). This ganglion contains only several hundred cell bodies (Fig. 79), which are comparatively large, clearly visible and readily accessible to investigation with intracellular micropipettes. It is possible to select cells (Y) within this ganglion that can be excited by either of two independent afferent pathways (X_1 and X_2; see Fig. 68). Stimulating electrodes are applied to the two connectives (Fig. 79) and one can then provide a weak test stimulus to an

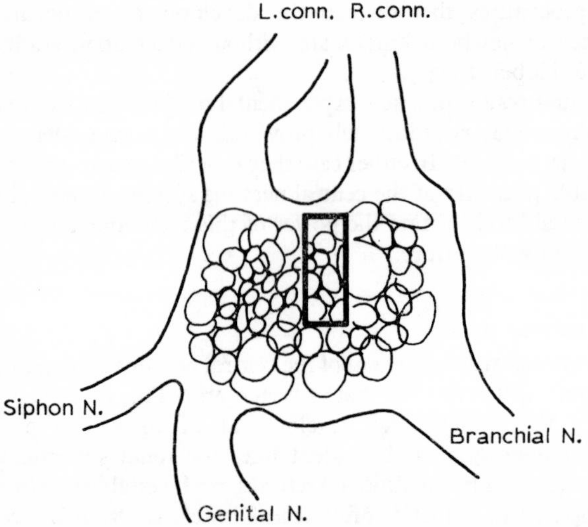

FIG. 79. Schematic view of the dorsal surface of the abdominal ganglion of *Aplysia depilans*. The area containing cells showing heterosynaptic facilitation is outlined. The connectives emerge from the upper corners of the ganglion, the nerves from the lower margin. Magnification approximately 20 ×.

(From Kandel & Tauc, 1965*a*, *J. Physiol.*, **181**, 1, Fig. 2.)

afferent pathway, X_1, of such a strength that it only produces a small excitatory post-synaptic potential in Y. The other afferent pathway, X_2, is used for the provision of stronger priming or conditioning stimuli, that are sufficient to cause a train of action potentials from the efferent cell, *Y*. Kandel and Tauc found a few cells for which a period of exposure to the priming stimulus, given together with or soon after the test stimulus (paired stimulation), resulted in a long-lasting facilitation of

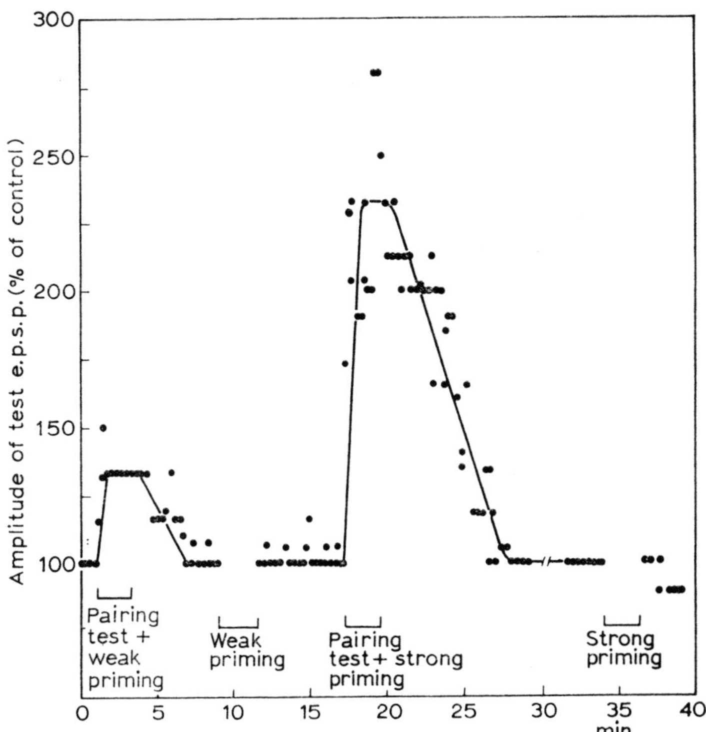

FIG. 80. Effects of paired and unpaired priming stimuli of differing efficacy. Graph illustrates four consecutive runs with the same test input. The first two runs were with a weak priming stimulus (a single shock producing a single spike). This priming stimulus was first paired with the test E.P.S.P. and subsequently presented alone. Note that the facilitation only occurred when the test input was paired with the priming stimulus. The next two runs were with a more effective priming stimulus (a train of 6/sec for 1 sec); the facilitation was greater than that with the weak priming stimulus and again the facilitation only occurred with pairing.

(From Kandel & Tauc, 1965*a*, *J. Physiol.*, **181**, 1, Fig. 7.)

the test pathway (the $X_1 Y$ synapses). "The maximum facilitation of the test PSP in these cells was usually about 100% and the facilitation declined over an average period of 9 min. and a maximum period of 20 min. after pairing" (Fig. 80). Unpaired stimulation did not produce

M

facilitation, nor did weak priming stimulation when given alone. Potentiation was more effective after a strong paired priming stimulus that produced multiple responses from Y, than after a weak one.

Among the minority of neurones exhibiting this form of heterosynaptic facilitation was the giant cell—one that is usually identifiable by its size and dark orange pigmentation. Unlike its smaller neighbours, however, this cell showed heterosynaptic facilitation following a period of unpaired conditioning. Neither cell type exhibited any change or conductivity in the test pathway, $X_1 Y$, when Y was caused to fire either by direct excitation through the intracellular electrode, or by stimulation of X_2 alone. Thus, the behaviour of this system appears to be different from that of cat's cerebral cortex discussed in Chapter 7. In the sea-slug, synaptic conductivity was not correlated with either y, or $\bar{x}y$—using the symbols of p. 145. Kandel & Tauc concluded that a presynaptic facilitation which increased the liberation of humoral transmitter by the test volleys was the factor responsible for the changes in conductivity that they observed. This would indicate a direct presynaptic effect of the X_2 afferent terminals upon the efficiency of the X_1 terminals, similar to that first described by Frank & Fuortes (1957) (see also Mendell & Wall, 1964). It would imply a positive correlation between conductivity and the frequency of more-or-less simultaneous discharge in X_1 and X_2, which could be written as $(x_1\ x_2)$, using the terminology of Chapter 7.

Tauc has examined a similar, relatively long-lasting, heterosynaptic inhibition which can be recorded in the same ganglion (Tauc, 1965). His results provide even more convincing evidence that the induced changes in synaptic conductivity have a presynaptic origin.

The neurophysiology of the sea-slug may seem to be a long way removed from that of the cat or dog. Nevertheless, *Aplysia* provide an elemental nervous system that is convenient for many types of experiment and can give relatively unambiguous answers to some important simple questions. It seems unlikely that these answers will prove irrelevant to an understanding of more complicated nervous systems.

Neural explants

I have stressed in the paragraphs above what is admittedly only one objective of comparative neurophysiology—namely, the search for a system of neurones of sufficient simplicity that the majority of factors governing its operation can be easily controlled. A promising alternative to this search would be to grow a nervous system according to a prearranged and simple 'wiring diagram', in such a way that all important elements are readily accessible. At present this cannot be done, but the recent publications of Crain & Bornstein leave little doubt that this objective will soon be attained. It is already possible to excise small

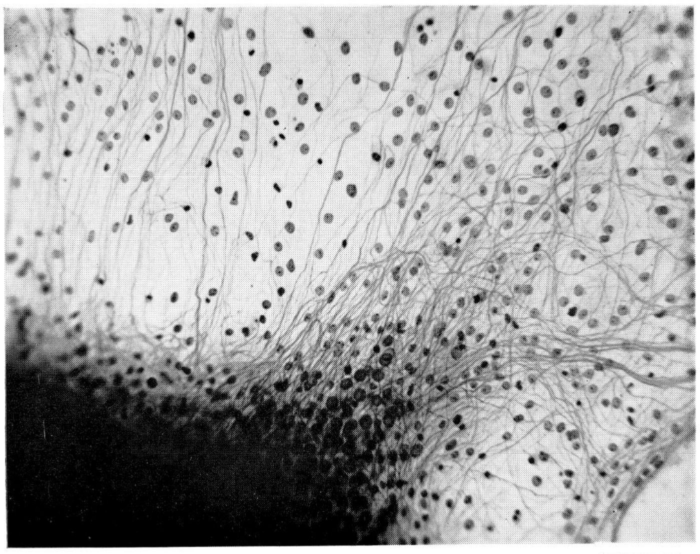

FIG. 82. Photomicrograph of mouse cerebral culture after three weeks *in vitro*. Pial edge of explant (lower left) showing numerous outgrowing neurites which emerge from fragment along with neuroglia cells (Bodian silver-impregnation). Calibration bar: 50 μ. (Kindly provided by Dr. S. M. Crain.)

pieces of cerebral cortex from the brain of newborn mammals and culture the explants *in vitro*. Crain & Bornstein (1964) describe the preparation of an explant from 1 to 5-day-old mouse cortex (Fig. 81); the

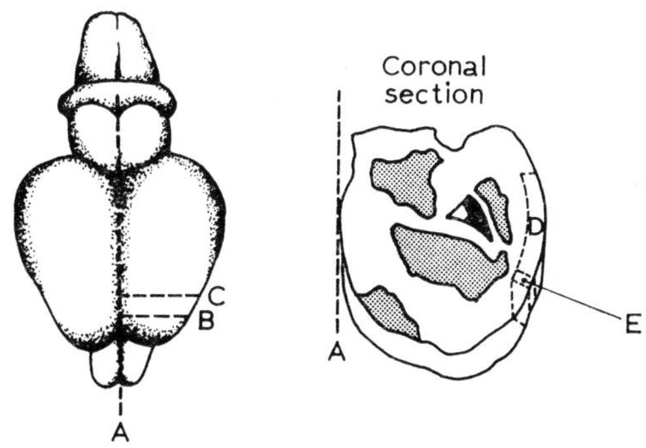

FIG. 81. Diagrammatic representation of a mouse brain showing the dissection followed to obtain the explants of cerebral cortex. The hemispheres are first separated by a cut along line *A*. A coronal section of the hemisphere, about 2 mm wide, is cut by sectioning along lines *B* and *C*. A wedge, *D*, is cut from the coronal section and this, in turn, is cut into segments (e.g. *E*) which are then explanted.
(From Crain & Bornstein, 1964, *Expl Neurol.*, **10**, 425, Fig. 1.)

explants they used measured roughly 2 × 1 × 0·5 mm and included cortex with some underlying white matter. The tissue was transferred to a cover-slip, covered with a thin layer of collagen gel and then fed with 2 drops of nutrient medium per week. The whole was kept in an atmosphere of 5% CO_2: 95% O_2. Provision was made for stimulating and recording through extracellular metal micro-electrodes of 10-25 μ tip diameter.

Such explants remain alive for 2 months or more, and during the first few days the transplanted cells differentiate into recognizable neurones, neuroglia, microglia and ependyma (Bornstein, 1963). There is no multiplication of cells, but during the first few days *in vitro* many neuritic processes grow out from the explanted fragment (Fig. 82); moreover, Crain & Bornstein (1964) have produced convincing functional evidence that new synaptic junctions are formed. During the first 2-3 days, stimulation of the white matter produces a single spike response of 2-3 msec duration from the overlying cortex. After the third or fourth day, the response to stimulation becomes more complex and progressively increases in duration. Indeed, the responses to single stimuli come to resemble in many ways the burst responses of cortex that has been neurologically isolated in the adult cat. (see Fig. 28 and pp. 62–65). The prolonged, irregular after-discharge that follows a single

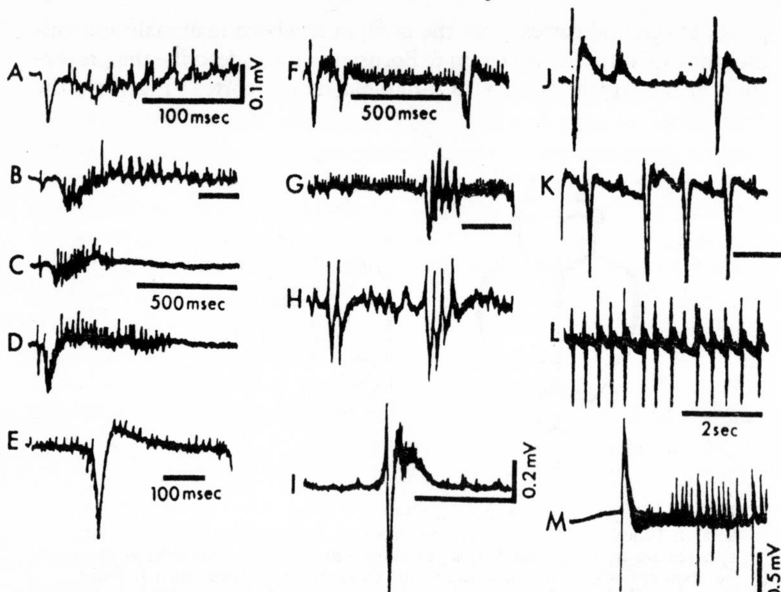

FIG. 83. Complex spike and slow-wave patterns in cultured neonatal cerebral cortex tissue after 14 days *in vitro*.

(*A–D*) Long-duration barrage responses to single stimulus applied about 200 μ from recording site. Note spike potentials superimposed on slow waves.

(*E–I*) Spontaneous slow waves with repetitive spikes.

(*J–L*) Successive sweeps showing much longer barrage response following single stimulus applied at beginning of record (*J*); note decrease in sweep rate in (*K*) and (*L*).

(*M*) Similar sequence at still slower sweep rate. Note sudden appearance of spikes more than 2 seconds after large, early-latency evoked potential.

(From Crain, 1964, *Neurological and Electroencephalographical Correlative Studies in Infancy*, Fig. 5; New York: Grune & Stratton.)

stimulus (Fig. 83 A-D) suggests that a network of self-reexciting neurones has been formed.

There is no doubt that such explants contain live cells and functional synapses. The extent to which these home-grown, miniature nervous systems emulate normal function in the parent animal has still to be worked out. It is interesting in this connection, however, to read that they can be given disseminated sclerosis. Apparently, the addition of serum from human cases of disseminated sclerosis produces a reversible demyelination within the explant (Bornstein & Crain, 1964).

The future usefulness of this new technique to neurophysiology, neuropharmacology and medicine is already apparent. Nevertheless, it is not yet possible to grow a small system of neurones with interconnecting synaptic junctions according to some prearranged and accessible pattern of cells. To do this it will be necessary to grow cultures in sheets of unicellular thickness—and this has so far proved impossible. Despite the present limitations of this method, one has to agree with Crain & Bornstein (1964) that this new line of investigation ". . . will become increasingly fruitful, as improvements in culture technique and in optical systems permit greater cytologic resolution during functional investigation of organized CNS networks *in vitro*". They conclude their paper by saying: "Although the structure and function of these tiny neuronally isolated explants are certainly altered in many respects, characteristic bioelectric activities are sufficiently preserved to warrant their use as a faithful model system to supplement *in situ* studies of nervous tissue. This experimental approach may permit close correlation of some of the bioelectric and cytological properties of CNS at a level unattainable in the living animal."

USEFUL RESEARCH

Despite its limitations, statistical neurophysiology has already made some contribution to one's understanding of function in the normal nervous system. Nevertheless, it is only one among many experimental techniques and I do not feel that its importance should be exaggerated; its current popularity and success should not be allowed to belittle the usefulness of entirely different methods. It seems to me that the danger of statistical techniques is one shared by all methods that employ complex apparatus. During recent decades, the preamplifier and oscilloscope have largely replaced the spring-myograph and smoked drum, and our present understanding of neural mechanisms is largely dependent upon these electronic instruments. At the same time, it has proved so easy to photograph the face of an oscilloscope that many worthy scientific observations have become buried in an avalanche of meaningless neural portraits. Statistical neurophysiology could present the same sort of threat to scientific progress, unless employed with greater caution than was the oscilloscope. Unfortunately, it is far easier to feed an electronic computer with action potentials and thus acquire a sheaf of graphs, than it is to devise a technique that answers a useful question in an unambiguous way.

While it is clear that a good experimental technique is one that provides results permitting a relatively small number of possible interpretations, it is less easy to define a 'useful' scientific question. Nevertheless, it seems important to attempt a definition, however inadequate the result, at a time when an ever-increasing fraction of every national income is being devoted to scientific research. Undoubtedly, the contemporary popularity of scientists in educational establishments, research institutions and industry is soundly based on the belief that sooner or later the results of science, however academic, raise the standard of living. Perhaps as a consequence of this partly justified public faith, the ambitions of scientists are not questioned as often as they should be. (Only two or three hundred years ago, I should have been burnt at the stake for activities which are now supported from the public purse; while my presently less-fortunate friends in the fine arts, would have lived comfortably under the wing of some rich benefactor!)

One way of defining a useful scientific pursuit is to pose a question that seems useless and then to examine its properties. For instance, I believe that it would be quite difficult to obtain a research grant in support of an investigation into 'The Relation between Intelligence in Cats and the Number of Hairs on their Tails'. There is no doubt that such a project would be feasible. Intelligence could be arbitrarily specified as performance of the animal when faced with a number of problem situations; the tail-skin could be anatomically defined in such a way that hair counts were estimated with little experimental error. Moreover, there is no *a priori* reason for believing that a relationship between these two measures does not exist. Suppose that a research grant were provided and that, after two or three years of painstaking study, a statistically significant correlation were established. What could the authors do with their results? They could publish their findings—but what next? I believe that a useful project must make intelligible intellectual contact with established scientific belief and must also lead to a new set of useful questions.

One might defend the 'useless' project of my example by pointing out that many scientific results that were once hard to believe or understand, have ultimately become an essential part of some accepted scientific creed. It is presumably such optimism that leads many authors to publish their results and leave the responsibility of interpretation and understanding to their weary readers. There is, after all, some evidence that undigested factual knowledge of this sort can occasionally prove useful to subsequent generations of scientists. Despite this, it seems to offer an uneconomical technique for the expansion of organized knowledge. The 'random project', which comes from nowhere and apparently leads nowhere, provides an expensive recipe for the acquisition of factual knowledge. The probability that results obtained in this way will become an essential part of structured understanding is too small.

My own working definition of a useful scientific project, runs somewhat as follows:

1. It should be possible to describe the project as a question or set of questions, the answer to which must be either 'yes' or 'no'. (This belittles the worthiness of such topics as 'The relation between heart

and respiratory rates during exercise': 'An investigation of rheumatoid arthritis'.)

2. It should be possible to define all of the words used in the questions set. ('Is the thalamic reticular system the site of consciousness' would not be an acceptable question.)
3. The project can only be useful if the answers to the questions set are accessible by contemporary techniques.
4. The value of a question is greatest when the number of interpretations allowed by the possible results of experiment is smallest.
5. The results should lead to an extension or modification of present scientific understanding; that is to say, the support or replacement of existing generalizations.
6. The resultant new or modified hypothesis should suggest a new set of useful scientific questions.

It is clear that the same demands cannot be made of applied research, in that applied science normally sets out to make use of existing knowledge for the solution of some social problem. The results of applied research are not expected to lead to new questions. Its technical merit must be measured by its success in solving a question set by the present needs of society. Its desirability, on the other hand, can never exceed the urgency with which society rates the problem set. If society is faced with more pressing problems, the value of research aimed at putting man on the moon is diminished.

It is easy to criticize the short list of criteria that I have suggested might be used as a crude gauge for the worthiness of research projects. There is no doubt that a rigid application of these requirements during the last century would have deprived contemporary science of some accidental but useful discoveries. If the reader quarrels with my measures of usefulness—as well he may—my main purpose will have been served. The assumption that all carefully made observations are of equal scienctific value will have been challenged.

Even scientific ambitions that are indisputably useful appear to be guided more by fashion than by the availability of novel techniques. The day of the 'Suppressor Band' is gone; the popularities of the 'Reticular System' and the 'Cell Assembly' are probably past their peaks; and it is not hard to predict that the limitations of statistical neurophysiology will soon become apparent. I suppose that fashion in science is the necessary result of a social structure in which each new generation of young scientists must appeal to the prejudices of their elders in order to obtain financial support. In making this comment, I am not, of course, implying that I know of any better system for the distribution of public money.

If any criticism were to be levelled at the accepted arrangements for the guidance of scientific effort, it would be that the mean age of granting committees is often too great. (In this context, perhaps age should be reckoned in years since the last independent publication!) But whatever the composition of granting committees, the responsibilities for the proper distribution of public resources will probably remain with 'established scientists'. Society has elected the latter to ensure a reasonable satisfaction of scientific ambition; it is just as important, however, that they should create a wide market of diverse demands. In this connection, it seems to me that the statesmen of science often spend too much of their time organizing and attending recurrent conferences, the main purpose of which is to tell us once again what we have already read.

It might prove rewarding to hold an occasional conference concerned with what we do not know. Some public discussion of ignorance that is masked by accepted terminology, some attempt to formulate useful questions that appear to be answerable by available techniques, might help to break the hold of fashion on neurophysiology.

REFERENCES

Adrian, E. D. (1936). The spread of activity in the cerebral cortex. *J. Physiol.*, **88,** 127–61.

Adrian, E. D. & Matthews, B. H. C. (1934). The Interpretation of potential waves in the cortex. *J. Physiol.*, **81,** 440–71.

Amassian, V. E., Berlin, J., Macy, J. & Waller, H. J. (1959). Simultaneous recording of the activities of several individual cortical neurones. *Ann. N.Y. Acad. Sci.*, **21,** 395–405.

Anderson, P. & Lømo, T. (1965). Excitation of hippocompal pyramidal cells by dendritic synapses. *J. Physiol.*, **181,** 39 *P.*

— (1950). The stability of a randomly assembled nerve-network. *Electroen. Neurophysiol.*, **2,** 471–82.

— (1952). Design for a brain. *C.N.S. Statistics*, p. 260. London: Chapman and Hall.

— (1966). Mathematical models and computer analysis of the function of the central nervous system. *A. Rev. Physiol.*, **28,** 89–106.

Averbach, E. & Sperling, G. (1960). Short term storage of information in vision. In *Symposium: Information theory*. ed. Cherry C. pp. 196–211. London: Butterworth.

Barlow, H. B. (1953). Summation and inhibition in the frog's retina. *J. Physiol.*, **119,** 69–88.

— (19
re
36
Barlow
sp
J.
Barlow
b
9,
Benne
w
Beurle
p
Bindm
b
fl
1
Birks,
er
Bishop
cı

ERRATA

Page 177, lines 8–15 should read:

Anderson, P. & Lømo, T. (1965). Excitation of hippocampal pyramidal cells by dendritic synapses. *J. Physiol.*, **181,** 39*P.*

Ashby, W. R. (1950). The stability of a randomly assembled nerve-network. *Electroen. Neurophysiol.*, **2,** 471–82.

— (1952). Design for a brain. *C.N.S. Statistics*, p. 260. London: Chapman and Hall.

— (1966). Mathematical models and computer analysis of the function of the central nervous system. *A. Rev. Physiol.*, **28,** 89–106.

BURNS: *The Uncertain Nervous System*

Bliss, T. V. P., Burns, B. D. & Uttley, A. M. (1968). Factors affecting the conductivity of pathways in the cerebal cortex. (In preparation.)

Bornstein, M. B. (1963). Morphological development of cultured mouse cerebral neocortex. *Trans. Ass. Am. Neur.*, 22–4.

Bornstein, M. B. & Crain, S. M. (1965). Functional studies of cultured brain tissues as related to "Demyelinative Disorders". *Science, N.Y.*, **148,** 1242–4.

Boyd, I. A. & Martin, A. R. (1956). The end-plate potential in mammalian muscle. *J. Physiol.*, **132,** 74–91.

Bradley, P. B. & Wolstencroft, J. H. (1964). Unit frequency meter. *J. Physiol.*, **170,** 2 *P.*

Brazier, M. A. B. (1949). The electrical fields at the surface of the head during sleep. *Electroen. Neurophysiol.*, **1,** 195–204.

— (1961). Recordings from large electrodes. *Meth. med. Res.*, **9,** 405–32.

Brazier, M. A. B. & Casby, J. U. (1952). Cross-correlation and auto-correlation studies of electroen-cephalographic potentials. *Electroen. Neurophysiol.*, **4,** 201–11.

Brindley, G. S. & Merton, P. A. (1960). The absence of position sense in the human eye. *J. Physiol.*, **153,** 127–30.

Brown, G. L. & Euler, U. S. von. (1938). The after-effects of a tetanus on mammalian muscle. *J. Physiol.*, **93,** 39–60.

Buller, A. J., Nicholls, J. G. & Strom G. (1953). Spontaneous fluctuations of excitability in the muscle spindle of the frog. *J. Physiol.*, **122,** 409–18.

Bures, J. & Buresova, D. (1956). A study on the metabolic nature and physiological manifestations of the spreading EEG depression of Leao. *Physiologia bohemoslov.*, **5,** 4–6.

Burns, B. D. (1951). Some properties of isolated cerebral cortex in the unanaesthetized cat. *J. Physiol.*, **112,** 156–75.

— (1956). The cause of reflex afterdischarge in the frog's spinal cord. *Can. J. Biochem. Physiol.*, **34,** 456–65.

— (1957). Electrophysiologic basis of normal and psychotic function. In *Psychotropic Drugs*, ed. Garattini & Ghetti, pp. 177–84. Amsterdam: Elsevier.

— (1958). *The Mammalian Cerebral Cortex*, p. 119. London: Edward Arnold.

— (1961). Use of extracellular microelectrodes. *Meth. med. Res.*, **9,** 354–80.

— (1963). The central control of respiratory movements. *Br. med. Bull.*, **19,** 7–9.

Burns, B. D., Ferch, W. & Mandl, G. (1965). A neurophysiological computer. *Electron. Engng*, **37,** 20–4.

Burns, B. D. & Grafstein, B. (1952). The function and structure of some neurones in the cat's cerebral cortex. *J. Physiol.*, **118,** 412–33.

Burns, B. D., Heron, W. & Grafstein, B. (1960). Responses of cerebral cortex to diffuse monocular and binocular stimulation. *Am. J. Physiol.*, **198,** 200–4.

Burns, B. D., Heron, W. & Pritchard, R. (1962). Physiological excitation of visual cortex in cat's unanaesthetized isolated forebrain. *J. Neurophysiol.*, **25,** 165–81.

Burns, B. D., Mandl, G. & Smith, G. K. (1963). An auto- and cross-correlator for digital information. *Electron. Engng*, **35,** 220–8.

Burns, B. D. & Pritchard, R. (1964). Contrast discrimination by neurones in the cat's visual cerebral cortex. *J. Physiol.*, **175,** 445–63.

Burns, B. D. & Pritchard, R. M. (1968). Cortical conditions for fused binocular vision. (In preparation.)

Burns, B. D. & Robson, J. G. (1960). 'Weightless' microelectrodes for recording extracellular unit action potentials from the central nervous system. *Nature, Lond.*, **186,** 246–7.

Burns, B. D. & Salmoiraghi, G. C. (1960). Repetitive firing of respiratory neurones during their burst activity. *J. Neurophysiol.*, **23,** 27–46.

Burns, B. D. & Smith, G. K. (1962). Transmission of information in the unanaesthetized cat's isolated forebrain. *J. Physiol.*, **164**, 238–51.

Buser, P., Borenstein, P. & Bruner, J. (1959). Etude des systeines "associatifis" visuels et anditifs chez le chat anesthesie an chloralose. *Electroen. Neurophysiol.*, **11**, 305–24.

Butler, T. C. (1950). Theories of general anaesthesia. In: *J. Pharmac. exp. Ther. Pharmac. Rev.* **2**, 121–60.

Ramon y Cajal, S. (1952–1955). *Histologie du Système Nerveux de l'homme et des vertebrés*. Madrid: Consejo Superior de Investigaciones Cientificas.

Campbell, E. J. M. & Howell, J. B. L. (1963). The sensation of breathlessness. *Br. med. Bull.*, **19**, 36–40.

Campbell, F. W., Robson, J. G. & Westheimer, G. (1959). Fluctuations of accommodation under steady viewing conditions. *J. Physiol.*, **145**, 579–94.

Campbell, F. W. & Westheimer, G. (1960). Dynamics of accommodation responses of the human eye. *J. Physiol.*, **151**, 285–95.

Camras, M. (1965). Information storage density. *C.N.S. Statistics IEEE Spectrum*, **2**, No. 7, 98–105.

Castillo, J. Del & Katz, B. (1954). Quantal components of the end-plate potential. *J. Physiol.*, **124**, 560–73.

Clark, A. D. (1931). Muscle counts of motor units: a study of innervation ratios. *Am. J. Physiol.*, **96**, 296–304.

Colonnier, M. (1964). The tangential organisation of the visual cortex. *J. Anat.*, **98**, 327–44.

Coombs, J. S., Curtis, D. R. & Eccles, J. C. (1957). The generation of impulses in motoneurones. *J. Physiol.*, **139**, 232–49.

Cornsweet, T. N. (1956). Determination of the stimuli for involuntary drifts and saccadic (flick) eye movements. *J. opt. Soc. Am.*, **46**, 987–93.

Costenbader, F. D. (1958). Principles and techniques of nonsurgical treatment. In *Strabismus Ophthalmic: Symposium II*, ed. Allen, J. H., pp. 312–24, 552. St. Louis: Mosby.

Cragg, E. G. & Temperley, H. N. V. (1954). The organisation of neurones: a cooperative analogy. *Electroen. Neurophysiol.*, **6**, 85–92.

Crain, S. M. (1964). Development of Bioelectric Activity During Growth of Neonatal Mouse Cerebral Cortex in Tissue Culture, pp. 12–26. New York: Grune and Stratton.

Crain, S. M. & Bornstein, M. B. (1964). Bioelectric activity of neonatal mouse cerebral cortex during growth and differentiation in tissue culture. *Expl Neurol.*, **10**, 425–50.

Daniel, P. M. & Whitteridge, D. (1961). The representation of the visual field on the cerebral cortex in monkeys. *J. Physiol.*, **159**, 203–21.

Dawson, G. D. (1947). Cerebral responses to electrical stimulation of peripheral nerve in man. *J. Neurol. Psychiat., Lond.*, **10**, 137–40.

— (1950). Human cortical responses to stimulation of peripheral nerves. *Br. med. Bull.*, **6**, 326–9.

— (1951). A summation technique for detecting small signals in a large irregular background. *J. Physiol.* **115**, 2 *P.*

— (1954). Summation technique for the detection of small evoked potentials. *Electroen. Neurophysiol.*, **6**, 65–84.

Dejong, D. & Burns, B. D. (1967). Parkinson's Disease—A random process. *Can. med. Ass. J.*, **97**, 49–56.

Descartes, R. (1664). *L'homme et un traiité de la formation du foetus*, p. 448. Paris: Charles Angot.

Ditchburn, R. W. (1956). Eye movements in relation to retinal action. In *Problems in contemporary optics*, pp. 609–23. Arcetri-Firenze: Istituto Nazionale di ottica.

Ditchburn, R. W. & Fender, D. H. (1955). The stabilized retinal image. *Optica Acta*, **2**, 128–33.

Ditchburn, R. W., Fender, D. H. & Mayne, S. (1959). Vision with controlled movements of the retinal image. *J. Physiol.*, **145**, 98–107.

Ditchburn, R. W. & Ginsborg, B. L. (1952). Vision with stabilized retinal image. *Nature, Lond.*, **170**, 36–7.

— — (1953). Involuntary eye movements during fixation. *J. Physiol.*, **119**, 1–17.

Durup, G. & Fessard, A. (1935). L'electroencephalogram de l'homme. *Ann. psychol.*, **36**, 1.

Eccles, J. C. (1953). *The Neurophysiological Basis of Mind*, p. 314. Oxford: Clarendon Press.

— (1957). *The Physiology of Nerve Cells*, p. 270. Baltimore: Johns Hopkins.

— (1964) *The Physiology of Synapses*, p. 316. Berlin: Springer Verlag.

Eccles, J. C., Anderson, P. & Løyning, Y. (1963). Recurrent inhibition in the hippocampus with identification of the inhibitory cell and its synapses. *Nature, Lond.*, **198**, 541–2.

Eccles, J. C., Fatt, P. & Koketsu, K. (1954). Cholinergic and inhibitory synapses in a pathway from motor axon collaterals to motor neurones. *J. Physiol.*, **126**, 524–62.

Eccles, J. C. & Kuffler, S. (1941). The endplate potential during and after the muscle spike potential. *J. Neurophysiol.*, **4**, 486–506.

Eccles, J. C. & McIntyre, A. K. (1953). The effects of disuse and of activity on mammalian spinal reflexes. *J. Physiol.*, **121**, 492–516.

Eccles, J. C. & O'Connor, W. J. (1939). Responses which nerve impulses evoke in mammalian striated muscles. *J. Physiol.*, **97**, 44–102.

Eccles, J. C. & Sherrington, C. S. (1930). Numbers and contraction-values of individual motor-units examined in some muscles of the limb. *Proc. R. Soc.* B., **106**, 326–57.

Eldred, E., Granit, R. & Merton, P. A. (1953). Supraspinal control of the muscle spindles and its significance. *J. Physiol.*, **122**, 498–523.

Evans, C. R. & Newman, E. A. (1964). Dreaming: An analogy from computers. *New Scientist*, **24**, 577–9.

Evans, E. F., Ross, H. F. & Whitfield, I. C. (1965). The spatial distribution of unit characteristic frequency in the primary auditory cortex of the cat. *J. Physiol.*, **179**, 238–47.

Farley, B. G. & Clark, W. A. (1960). Activity in networks of neurone-like elements. In *Proc. 4th London Symposium on Information theory*, pp. 242–51, 476. London: Butterworth.

Fatt, P. (1950). The electromotive action of acetylcholine at the motor endplate. *J. Physiol.*, **111**, 408–22.

— (1957*a*). Electric potentials occurring around a neurone during its antidromic activation. *J. Neurophysiol.*, **20**, 27–60.

— (1957*b*). Sequence of events in synaptic activation of a motor neurone *J. Neurophysiol*, **20**, 61–80.

— (1959). Skeletal neuromuscular transmission. In *American Physiological Society. Handbook of Physiology. Section* 1, *Neurophysiology*, Vol. **1**, 199–214.

Fatt, P. & Katz, B. (1950). Some observations on biological noise. *Nature, Lond.*, **166**, 597–8.

Fatt, P. & Katz, B. (1951). An analysis of the end-plate potential recorded with an intracellular electrode. *J. Physiol.*, **115**, 320–70.

— — (1952). Spontaneous subthreshold activity at motor nerve endings. *J. Physiol.*, **117**, 109–28.

Feigenbaum, E. A. & Feldman, J. (1963). *Computers and Thought*, p. 535. New York and Maidenhead: McGraw-Hill.

Feller, W. (1950). *Introduction to probability Theory and its Applications*, p. 419. New York and London: John Wiley.

Firth, D. R. (1966). Interspike interval fluctuations in the crayfish stretch receptor. *Biophys. J.*, **6**, 201–15.

Fitzhugh, R. (1957). The statistical detection of threshold signals in the retina. *J. gen. Physiol.*, **40**, 925–48.

Forbes, A. (1929). The mechanism of reaction. *The foundations of experimental psychology*, ed. Murchison, C., pp. 128–68, 907: Worc. Mass: Clark. Univ. Press.

Foster, M. (1901). *Lectures on the History of Physiology during the Sixteenth Seventeenth and Eighteenth Centuries*, p. 310. Cambridge: University Press.

Frank, K. & Fuortes, M. G. F. (1956). Stimulation of spinal motoneurones with intracellular electrodes. *J. Physiol.*, **134**, 451–70.

— — (1957). Presynaptic and post-synaptic inhibition of monosynaptic reflexes. *Fedn Proc.*, **16**, 39–40.

Gerstein, G. L. & Kiang, N. Y. -S. (1960). An approach to the quantitative analysis of electro-physiological data from single neurons. *Biophys. J.*, **1**, 15–28.

Glees, P. & Cole, J. (1950). Recovery of skilled motor functions after small repeated lesions of motor cortex in macaque. *J. Neurophysiol.*, **13**, 137–48.

Gloor, P. (1963). Identification of inhibitory neurones in the hippocampus. *Nature, Lond.*, **199**, 699–700.

Goodman, L. S. & Gilman, A. (1965). *Pharmacological Basis of Therapeutics*, p. 1785. New York: Macmillan. London: Collier-Macmillan.

Granit, R. (1955). *Receptors and Sensory Perception*, p. 369. Oxford: University Press.

Gray, J. A. B. (1959). Initiation of impulses at receptors, pp. 123–46. In *Handbook of Physiology, Section 1: Neurophysiology*, Vol. 1, p. 779. Washington: Amer. Physiol. Soc.

Haber, E., Kohn, K. W., Ngai, S. H., Holaday, D. A. & Wang, S. C. (1957). Localization of spontaneous respiratory neuronal activities in the medulla oblongata of the cat: A new location of the expiratory center. *Am. J. Physiol.*, **190**, 350–5.

Hagiwara, S. (1954). Analysis of interval fluctuation of the sensory nerve impulse. *Jap. J. Physiol.*, **4**, 234–40.

Hammond, P. H., Merton, P. A. & Sutton, G. G. (1956). Nervous gradation of muscular contraction. *Br. med. Bull.*, **12**, 214–18.

Hartline, H. K. (1938). The response of single optic nerve fibres of the vertebrate eye to illumination of the retina. *Am. J. Physiol.*, **121**, 400–15.

Hebb, D. O. (1949). *The Organization of Behaviour*, p. 335. New York and London: John Wiley.

Heymans, G. (1896). Quantitative Untersuchungen uber das "optische Paradoxon". *Z. Psychol.*, **9**, 221–55.

Holmes, O. & Houchin, Jane. (1966). Units in the cerebral cortex of the anaesthetized rat and the correlations between their discharges. *J. Physiol.*, **187**, 651–71.

Hubel, D. H. (1963). Integrative processes in central pathways of the cat. *J. opt. Soc. Am.*, **53**, 58–66.

Hubel, D. H. & Wiesel, T. N. (1959). Receptive fields of single neurones in the cat's striate cortex. *J. Physiol.*, **148,** 579–91.

— — (1960). Receptive fields of optic nerve fibres in the spider monkey. *J. Physiol.*, **154,** 572–80.

— — (1961). Integrative action in the cat's lateral geniculate body. *J. Physiol.*, **155,** 385–98.

— — (1962). Receptive fields, binocular interaction and functional architecture in the cat's visual cortex. *J. Physiol.*, **160,** 106–54.

— — (1963*a*). Shape and arrangement of columns in cat's striate cortex. *J. Physiol.*, **165,** 559–68.

— — (1963*b*). Receptive fields of cells in striate cortex of very young, visually inexperienced kittens. *J. Neurophysiol.*, **26,** 994–1002.

— — (1965*a*). Receptive fields and functional architecture in two non-striate visual areas (18 × 19) of the cat. *J. Neurophysiol.*, **28,** 229–89.

— — (1965*b*). Binocular interaction in striate cortex of kittens reared with artificial squint. *J. Neurophysiol.*, **28,** 1041–59.

Hunt, C. C. (1951). The reflex activity of mammalian small-nerve fibres. *J. Physiol.*, **115,** 456–69.

Hunt, C. C. & Kuno, M. (1959). Background discharge and evoked responses of spinal interneurones. *J. Physiol.*, **147,** 364–84.

Jacobsen, C. F. (1932). Influence of motor and premotor area lesions upon the retention of skilled movement in monkeys and chimpanzees. *Proc. Ass. Res. Nerv. Ment. Dis.*, **13,** 225–47.

Jasper, H. H. Ricci, G. & Doane, B. (1960). Microelectrode analysis of cortical cell discharge during avoidance conditioning in the monkey. In *Moscow Colloquium on electroencephalography of higher nervous activity*, ed. H. H. J. & G. D. Smirnov. *Electroen. Neurophysiol.*, Suppl. 13.

Jasper, H. & Shagass, C. (1941*a*). Conditioning occipital alpha rhythm in man. *J. exp. Psychol.*, **28,** 373–88.

— — (1941*b*). Conscious time judgement related to conditioned time intervals and voluntary control of alpha rhythm. *J. exp. Psychol.*, **28,** 503–8.

Jouvet, M. & Hernandez-Peon, R. (1957). Mecanismes neurophysiologiques concernant l'habituation, l'attention et le conditionnement. *Electroen. Neurophysiol.*, Suppl. 6, 39–49.

Kandel, E., Frazier, W. & Coggershall, R. (1966). Opposite synaptic actions mediated by different branches of an identifiable interneuron in *Aplysia. Fed. Proc.*, **25,** 270.

Kandel, E. R. & Tauc, L. (1964). Mechanism of prolonged heterosynaptic facilitation. *Nature, Lond.*, **202,** 145–7.

— — (1965*a*). Heterosynaptic facilitation in neurones of the abdominal ganglion of *Aplysia depilans. J. Physiol.*, **181,** 1–27.

— — (1965*b*). Mechanism of heterosynaptic facilitation in the giant cell of the abdominal ganglion of *Aplysia depilans. J. Physiol.*, **181,** 28–47.

Katz, B. (1962). The transmission of impulses from nerve to muscle and the subcellular unit of synaptic action. (Croonian lecture.) *Proc. R. Soc.* B., **155,** 455–77.

Kolers, P. A. & Rosner, B. S. (1960). On visual masking (metacontrast): dichoptic observation. *Am. J. Psychol.*, **73,** 2–21.

Krauskopf, J., Cornsweet, T. N. & Riggs, L. A. (1960). Analysis of eye movements during monocular and binocular fixation. *J. opt. Soc. Am.*, **50,** 572–8.

Krnjevic, K. (1965). Actions of drugs on single neurones in the cerebral cortex. *Br. med. Bull.*, **21,** 10–14.

Krnjevic, K., Randic, Mirjana & Straughan, D. W. (1966*a*). An inhibitory process in the cerebral cortex. *J. Physiol.*, **184,** 16–48.

— — — — (1966*b*). Nature of a cortical inhibitory process. *J. Physiol.*, **184,** 49–77

Kuffler, S. W. (1943). Specific excitability of the endplate region in normal and denervated muscle. *J. Neurophysiol.*, **6,** 99–110.

— (1953). Discharge patterns and functional organization of mammalian retina. *J. Neurophysiol.*, **16,** 37–68.

Kuffler, S. W., Fitzhugh, R. & Barlow, H. B. (1957). Maintained activity in the cat's retina in light and darkness. *J. gen. Physiol.*, **40,** 683–702.

Kuffler, S. W. & Hunt, C. C. (1952). The mammalian small-nerve fibres, a system for efferent nervous regulation of muscle spindle discharge. *Res. Publs Ass. Res. nerv. ment. Dis.*, **30,** 24–47.

Kuffler, S. W., Hunt, C. C. & Quilliam, J. P. (1951). Function of medullated small-nerve fibres in mammalian ventral roots: Efferent muscle spindle innervation. *J. Neurophysiol.*, **14,** 29.

Larrabee, M. G. & Bronk, D. W. (1938). Persistent discharge from sympathetic ganglion cells following preganglionic stimulation. *Proc. Soc. exp. Biol., N.Y.*, **38,** 921–2.

Lashley, K. S. (1924). Studies of cerebral function in learning. V. The retention of motor habits after destruction of the so called motor area in primates. *Archs Neurol. Psychiat.*, Chicago, **12,** 249–76.

— (1929). Brain Mechanisms and Intelligence, p. 186. Dover: New York; London: Constable (1963).

— (1950). Physiological mechanisms in animal behaviour in search of the engram. *S.E.B. Symposia*, **IV,** 454–83.

Lettvin, J. Y., Maturana, H. R., McCulloch, W. S. & Pitts, W. H. (1959). What the frog's eye tells the frog's brain. *Proc. Inst. Radio Engrs*, **47,** No. 11, 1940–51.

Lewis, T. (1925). *The Mechanism and Graphic Registration of the Heart Beat*, p. 529. London: Shaw Pub.

Li, Choh-Luh (1959). Cortical intracellular potentials and their response to strychnine. *J. Neurophysiol.*, **22,** 436–50.

— (1961). Cortical intracellular synaptic potentials. *J. cell. comp. Physiol.*, **58,** 153–67.

Ling, G. & Gerard, R. W. (1949). Normal membrane potential of frog sartorius fibres. *J. cell. comp. Physiol.*, **34,** 383–96.

Lloyd, D. P. C. (1949). Post-tetanic potentiation of response in monosynaptic reflex pathways of the spinal cord. *J. gen. Physiol.*, **33,** 147–70.

McCulloch, W. S. & Pitts, W. (1943). A logical calculus of the ideas imminent in nervous activity. *Bull. math. Biophys.*, **5,** 115–33.

McIlroy, M. B., Marshall, R. & Christie, R. V. (1954). The work of breathing in normal subjects. *Clin. Sci.*, **13,** 127–36.

MacIntosh, F. C. & Oborin, P. E. (1953). Release of acetylcholine from intact cerebral cortex. *Abstr. XIX int. physiol. Congr.*, 580–1.

Mandl, G. (1968). Localization of visual patterns by cat's cerebral cortex. (In preparation.)

Martin, A. R. & Branch, C. L. (1958). Spontaneous activity of Betz cells in cats with midbrain lesions. *J. Neurophysiol.*, **21,** 368–79.

Matthews, P. B. C. (1964). Muscle spindles and their motor control. *Physiol. Rev.*, **44,** 219–88.

Maturana, H. R. & Frenk, S. (1963). Directional movement and horizontal edge detectors in the pigeon retina. *Science, N.Y.*, **142,** 977–99.

Maturana, H. R., Lettvin, J. Y., McCulloch, W. S. & Pitts, W. H. (1960). Anatomy and physiology of vision in the frog (*Rana pipiens*). *J. gen. Physiol.*, **43**, 129–76.

Mendell, L. M. & Wall, P. (1964). Presynaptic hyperpolarization: a role for fine afferent fibres. *J. Physiol.*, **172**, 274–94.

Merton, P. A. (1950). Significance of the silent period of muscles. *Nature, Lond.*, **166**, 733–4.

Milner, P. (1957). The cell assembly: Mark II. *Psychol. Rev.*, **64**, 242–52.

Milsum, J. H. (1966). *Biological Control Systems Analysis*, p. 466. New York and London: McGraw-Hill.

Minsky, M. (1961*a*). A selected descriptor-indexed bibliography to the literature on artificial intelligence. *IRE Transactions on human factors in electronics*, Vol. HFE-2, No. 1, 39–55.

— (1961*b*). Steps toward artificial intelligence. *Proc. Inst. Radio Engrs*, **49**, No. 1, 8–30.

Mitchell, J. F. (1963). The spontaneous and evoked release of acetylcholine from the cerebral cortex. *J. Physiol.*, **165**, 98–116.

Monro, A. (1763). *The Anatomy of the Human Bones, Nerves and Lacteal Sac and Duct*. 8th edn. Edinburgh: Hamilton & Balfour.

Morrell, F. (1961). Electrophysiological contributions to the neural basis of learning. *Physiol. Rev.*, **41**, 443–94.

Morrel, F. & Jasper, H. H. (1956). Electrographic studies of the formation of temporary connections in the brain. *Electroen. Neurophysiol.*, **8**, 201.

Mountcastle, V. B. (1957). Modality and topographic properties of single neurons of cat's somatic sensory cortex. *J. Neurophysiol.*, **20**, 408–34.

Mountcastle, V. B., Davies, P. W. & Berman, A. L. (1957). Response properties of neurons of cat's somatic sensory cortex to peripheral stimuli. *J. Neurophysiol.*, **20**, 374–407.

Nelson, J. R. (1959). Single unit activity in medullary respiratory centers of cat. *J. Neurophysiol.*, **22**, 590–8.

Ogle, K. N. (1950). *Researches in Binocular Vision*, p. 345. Philadelphia: Saunders.

O'Leary, J. L. & Bishop, G. H. (1938). Margins of the optically excitable cortex in the rabbit. *Archs Neurol. Psychiat., Lond.*, **40**, 482–99.

Pavlov, I. (1927). *Conditioned Reflexes*, p. 430. London: Milford.

Pearson, K. (1900). *The Grammar of Science*, 2nd edn., p. 548. London: Black.

Penfield, W. G. & Erickson, T. C. (1941). *Epilepsy and Cerebral Localization*, p. 212. Springfield, Illinois. C. C Thomas.

Phillips, C. G. (1959). Actions of antidromic pyramidal volleys on single Betz cells in the cat. *Q. Jl exp. Physiol.*, **44**, 1–25.

Pinsky, C. and Burns, B. D. (1962). Production of epileptiform afterdischarges in cat's cerebral cortex. *J. Neurophysiol.*, **25**, 359–79.

Plumb, G. O. (1965). Pulse height analyser for electrophysiology. *J. Physiol.*, **179**, 16 *P*.

Poggio, G. F. & Vierstein, L. J. (1964). Time series analysis of impulse sequences of thalamic somatic sensory neurons. *J. Neurophysiol.*, **27**, 517–45.

Powell, T. P. S. & Mountcastle, V. B. (1959). Some aspects of the functional organization of the cortex of the postcentral syrus of the monkey: a correlation of findings obtained in a single unit analysis with cytoarchitecture. *Johns Hopkins Hosp. Bull.*, **105**, 133–62.

Pritchard, R. M. (1958). Visual illusions viewed as stabilized retinal usages. *J. exp. Psychol.*, **10**, 77–81.

Pritchard, R. M. & Heron, W. (1960). Small eye movements of the cat. *Can. J. Psychol.*, **14**, 131–7.

Pritchard, R. M., Heron, W. & Hebb, D. O. (1960). Visual perception approached through the method of stabilized images. *Can. J. Psychol.*, **14**, 63–73.

Provins, K. A. (1958). The effect of peripheral nerve block on the appreciation and execution of finger movements. *J. Physiol.*, **143**, 55–67.

Ratliff, F. & Riggs, L. A. (1950). Involuntary motions of the eye during monocular fixation. *J. exp. Psychol.*, **40**, 687–701.

Riggs, L. A. & Niehl, E. W. (1960). Eye movements recorded during convergence and divergence. *J. opt. Soc. Am.*, **50**, 913–20.

Riggs, L. A., Ratliff, F., Cornsweet, J. C. & Cornsweet, T. N. (1953). The disappearance of steadily fixated visual test objects. *J. opt. Soc. Am.*, **43**, 495–501.

Robson, J. G., Burns, B. D. & Welt, P. J. L. (1960). The effect of inhaling dilute nitrous oxide upon recent memory and time estimation. *Can. Anaesth. Soc. J.*, **7**, 399–410.

Rodieck, R. W., Kiang, N. Y.-S. & Gerstein, G. L. (1962). Some quantitative methods for the study of spontaneous activity of single neurons. *Biophys. J.*, **2**, 351–68.

Rossi, G. (1927). Asimmetrie toniche posturali, ed asimmetrie motorie. *Archo Fisiol.*, **25**, 146–57.

Ruch, T. C. (1961). Somatic sensation. In *Neurophysiology*, ed. Ruch, T. C. & Patton, H. D., pp. 300–22. Philadelphia: Saunders.

Salmoiraghi, G. C. & Burns, B. D. (1960). Localization and patterns of discharge of respiratory neurones in brain-stem of cat. *J. Neurophysiol.*, **23**, 2–13.

Salmoiraghi, G. C. & Steiner, F. A. (1963). Acetylcholine sensitivity of cat's medullary neurons. *J. Neurophysiol.*, **26**, 581–97.

Schaefer, H. & Haass, P. (1939). Uber einen lokalen Erregunsstrom an der Motorischen Endplatte. *Pflügers Arch. ges. Physiol.* **242**, 364–81.

Sears, T. A. (1964). Some properties and reflex connections of respiratory motoneurones of the cat's thoracic spinal cord. *J. Physiol.*, **175**, 386–403.

Sherrington, C. (1940). *Man on his Nature*, p. 413. London: Cambridge Univ. Press.

Sholl, D. A. (1953). Dendritic organization in the neurons of the visual and motor cortices of the cat. *J. Anat.*, **87**, 387–407.

— (1956). *The Organization of the Cerebral Cortex*, p. 125. London: Methuen.

Smith, D. R. & Smith, G. K. (1965). A statistical analysis of the continual activity of single cortical neurones in the cat unanaesthetized isolated forebrain. *Biophys. J.*, **5**, 47–74.

Smith, G. K. & Burns, B. D. (1960). A biological interval analyser. *Nature, Lond.*, **187**, 512–13.

Sperry, R. W. (1947). Cerebral regulation of motor coordination in monkeys following multiple transection of sensorimotor cortex. *J. Neurophysiol.*, **10**, 275–94.

Sperry, R. W., Miner, Nancy & Myers, R. E. (1955). Visual pattern perception following subpial slicing and tantalum wire implantations in the visual cortex. *J. comp. physiol. Psychol.*, **48**, 50–8.

Spinelli, D. N. (1966). Visual receptive fields in the cat's retina: complications. *Science, N.Y.*, **152**, 1768–9.

Stark, L. (1959). Stability, oscillations and noise in the human pupil servo-mechanism. *Proc. Inst. Radio Engrs*, **47**, No. 11, 1925–39.

Stark, L., Campbell, F. W. & Atwood, J. (1958). Pupil unrest; an example of noise in a biological servo mechanism. *Nature, Lond.*, **182**, 857–8.

Stark, L., Kupfer, C. & Young, L. R. (1965). Physiology of the visual control system. *NASA Contractor Report*, CR–238, pp. 88.

Summerfeld, A. & Steinberg, H. (1957). Reducing interference in forgetting. *Q. Jl exp. Psychol.*, **9**, 146–54.

Svaetichin, G. (1951). Analysis of action potentials from single spinal ganglion cells. *Acta physiol. scand.*, **24**, Suppl. 86, 23–57.

Tauc, L. (1965). Presynaptic inhibition in the abdominal ganglion of *Aplysia. J. Physiol.*, **181**, 282–307.

Thesleff, S. (1960). Effects of motor innervation on the chemical sensitivity of skeletal muscle. *Physiol. Rev.*, **40**, 734–52.

Torre, M. (1953). Nombre ex dimensions des unites motrices dans les muscles extrinsèques de l'oeil et, en général, dans les muscles squélettiques reliés à des organes de sens. *Schweizer Arch. Neurol. Psychiat.*, **72**, 362–76.

Tunturi, A. R. (1950). Physiological determination of the arrangement of the afferent connections to the middle ectosylvian auditory area in the dog. *Am. J. Physiol.*, **162**, 489–502.

Uttley, A. M. (1954). The classification of signals in the nervous system. *Electroen. Neurophysiol.*, **6**, 479–94.

— (1956). A theory of the mechanism of learning based on the computation of conditional probabilities. *Proc. 1st Int. Congr. on Cybernetics. Namur.* Paris: Gauthier-Villars.

Wall, P. D. (1965). Impulses originating in the region of dendrites. *J. Physiol.*, **180**, 116–33.

Walshe, F. M. R. (1948). *Critical Studies in Neurology*, p. 256. Edinburgh: Livingstone.

Walter, W. Grey (1953). *The Living Brain*, p. 216. London: Duckworth.

Werner, H. (1935). Studies on contour. I. Qualitative analysis. *Am. J. Psychol.*, **47**, 40–64.

Weymouth, F. W. (1958). Visual sensory units and the minimal angle of re-solutions. *Am. J. Ophthal.*, **46**, 102–13.

Wiesel, T. N. & Hubel, D. H. (1963). Single cell responses in striate cortex of kittens deprived of vision in one eye. *J. Neurophysiol.*, **26**, 1003–17.

— — (1965*a*). Comparison of the effects of unilateral and bilateral eye closure on cortical unit responses in kittens. *J. Neurophysiol.*, **28**, 1029–40.

— — (1965*b*). Extent of recovery from the effects of visual deprivation in kittens. *J. Neurophysiol.*, **28**, 1060–72.

Woldring, S. & Dirken, M. N. J. (1951). Unit activity in bulbar respiratory centre. *J. Neurophysiol.*, **14**, 211–25.

Wright, E. B. (1954). Effect of Mephenesin and other 'Depressants' on spinal cord transmission in frog and cat. *Am. J. Physiol.*, **179**, 390–401.

Yarbus, A. L. (1957). On the perception of an image fixed relative to the retina. *Biofizika*, **2**, 703–12.

Young, J. Z. (1964). *A Model of the Brain*, p. 348. Oxford: Clarendon.

AUTHOR INDEX

SUBJECT INDEX